Trilogy

*How to help the Mind, Body & Spirit
survive Mouth, Head & Neck Cancer*

Carol Dunstone and Ann Bennett

Bloomington, IN 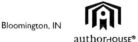 Milton Keynes, UK

authorHOUSE®

AuthorHouse™
1663 Liberty Drive, Suite 200
Bloomington, IN 47403
www.authorhouse.com
Phone: 1-800-839-8640

AuthorHouse™ UK Ltd.
500 Avebury Boulevard
Central Milton Keynes, MK9 2BE
www.authorhouse.co.uk
Phone: 08001974150

First published by AuthorHouse 10/13/2006

ISBN: 1-4259-5958-X (sc)

Printed in the United States of America
Bloomington, Indiana

This book is printed on acid-free paper.

Contents

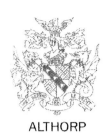

ALTHORP

17 June 2006

Dear Ann and Carol

Having had four grandparents who died from cancer and a mother who has happily recovered from a bout of it, I am all too aware of the devastation and trauma it can cause. I hope that this book can help cancer sufferers find complementary treatments in their battle with this terrible disease.

I wish you both every luck with your work.

Best wishes

Countess Spencer

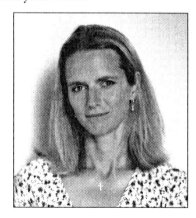

The Stables, Althorp, Northampton NN7 4HQ
Tel: +44 (0)1604 770107 Fax: +44 (0)1604 770042
e-mail: mail@althorp.com www.althorp.com

Acknowledgements

CAROL AND ANN would like to thank everyone who helped them throughout their journeys from diagnosis to recovery. They especially thank their families for their constant support:

Bunny; Carol's children, Alastair, Clare and James Kimbell; and her sisters, *Inga Sutton* and *Judy Shephard. Michael; Ann's son Mark;* and her sister, *Sarah Erickson.*

They also thank their friends for their support throughout, those who contributed recipes and all those named specialists who contributed articles. And they send special thanks to their Consultants and Medical teams.

Finally they thank all those involved in helping to produce this book: *Roger Wilkin, Eline Armstrong, Eugene Murray, Elsa Christie, Elke Pollard, Fiona Cannon, Roger Brown, 'Bazzerooni', Anne Hicks,* and their editor *Tony Boullemier.*

They would like to express thanks to *Countess Spencer* for writing the foreword and to World Cancer Research Fund for their interest and support.

INTRODUCTION

The Authors

CAROL DUNSTONE is a ceramic artist and had a full-time career until cancer of the mouth was diagnosed in 1998 at the age of 54.

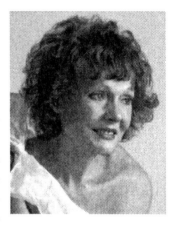

She lives in Northamptonshire with her husband, Brian, known as Bunny. She is the mother of three grown-up children and has four grandchildren. Her ceramic art continues and she works at home in her own studio along with Bunny who is a sculptor. Her interests include painting, reading, walking the dogs and family life.

She was making a good recovery from her illness when in 2001 she helped set up FACEFAX, a support group for head and neck cancer patients. There she met Ann Bennett and together they discussed how they could use their own experiences to collate information and provide tips and suitable cooking recipes for fellow patients and their families.

ANN BENNETT was born in Wiltshire and now lives in Northampton. She is married to Michael and has a 31-year-old son Mark. Her interests include entertainment, travel and reading.

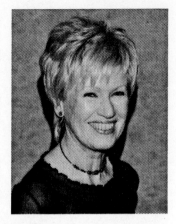

For many years she worked in the business world and in advertising but in 1993 decided to pursue her interest in complementary therapies and trained as an Advanced Reiki practitioner. She became a Full Healer Member with the National Federation of Spiritual Healers and went on to qualify as an Advanced Hypnotherapist and Hypno-healer. She has incorporated all three therapies in her practice.

She was 56 when she was diagnosed with mouth cancer in 2004. Eight months after her operation she met Carol Dunstone when she attended her first FACEFAX meeting. Together they decided to write this book to help fellow patients. The idea developed from their own individual journeys to include therapies, referral systems, and other helpful guidelines.

CHAPTER ONE

How FACEFAX started

*"Being told you have cancer or that your cancer
has returned or can't be cured, can leave
you feeling shocked, upset and very isolated.
There are so many feelings to deal
with and it can be a very confusing and
distressing time."*
– the Macmillan Cancer Line.

THE FACEFAX support group was first established in Northampton in June 2001 when it became apparent that many patients with mouth, head and neck cancer were not getting enough support on their journeys towards recovery.

When Carol Dunstone mentioned to her consultant Mr Clive Pratt that there seemed to be a lack of immediate contact and backup for patients like herself, he agreed. He suggested that she meet another patient named Valerie Johal who was recovering from mouth cancer. When she and Carol met, they found their experiences gave them a close bond.

They began meeting other patients about once a month at Northampton General Hospital with Sister Jane Bradley acting as facilitator. Their aim was to provide information and support to patients and carers and as the group grew, it was registered as a charity, The FACEFAX Association.

The association's main aim is to increase public and professional awareness of these cancers on a national scale and its intention is to become the umbrella organisation for a national network of support groups. More details can be found at the back of this book.

Anne Hicks now acts as the FACEFAX facilitator. She gives up much of her time listening to patients' problems and is always full of advice. The group regards her as indispensable.

A Unique Link

By Anne Hicks, Maxillofacial Clinical Nurse Specialist, Northampton General Hospital

MY patients are all undergoing treatment for head and neck cancer and since the diagnosis usually comes out of the blue, it is liable to leave them in a complete state of shock. But I will be present at the point of diagnosis and will be their point of contact in the hospital throughout their treatment.

I ensure that my patients and their loved ones get information about their planned treatment and offer emotional support as required. I encourage them to ask questions and discuss the life-changing experience they are having.

Verbal information is supported by a written information pack and given over two or three 45-minute consultations. It is important that patients and their loved ones understand all the treatment options and give their informed consent. Every patient will require different levels of information given at their own pace. As doctors and nurses we know that too much information given too soon after a diagnosis of cancer will not be understood, leading to problems later in the recovery process.

I manage all wounds following surgery and take part in the review process in conjunction with my medical colleagues. Consequently, the relationship with my patients will hopefully last at least five years.

I am chairman of FACEFAX and also facilitate the FACEFAX support group meetings held in Northampton. Only a small percentage of my patients attend regularly but those who do are so full of energy and enthusiasm that the meetings are exhausting.

We actively promote awareness of head, neck, mouth and face cancer and I am proud to say that the meetings are a very positive experience for everyone, whatever stage of the treatment process they are in. The people who attend are from all walks of life and a variety of ages, but with a life changing experience in common. They each have a unique story to tell and hold a wealth of information that I am able to learn from.

CHAPTER TWO

Carol's Story

*Her son Alastair recalls
how it all began*

"SO IT'S cancer then." I knew as soon as I saw the look on Bunny's face that the news wasn't good. I was on the front steps at Target where I used to work, and Bunny put a fatherly arm round me and took me outside to let me know the news about Mum's biopsy.

I don't remember much more than that. We must have talked about it and I remember my old boss, a close friend of Bunny's, asking if there was anything he could do and being very supportive. I had no idea what was going to happen next.

Mum and Bunny persuaded me to go ahead with my trip to Australia with a couple of friends. "It's not a big op, everything will be fine," they said, so off I went.

I'd just split up with a long time girlfriend, and was looking forward to letting my hair down away from it all for a few days. I spent a couple of weeks partying up the East Coast of Australia from Sydney to Cairns until the night before Mum's op. Then I was in Port Douglas, with Ann and Ian Black, family friends who knew Mum well and understood the situation. They were great, really supportive and kept a quiet eye on me, until I got the plane back to the UK.

I remember seeing Mum for the first time. Bunny, my sister Clare and brother James who had been there all along told me how much better she now looked but I was quietly horrified when I saw her. A tracheostomy, switches, tubes and monitors everywhere. I remember putting on a brave face, and sitting down by the bed. Mum couldn't talk to start with and communicated using a 'Point Card' that her sister Judy had made for her.

Apparently she was through the worst and had had a really rough time while I was in Australia, in and out of Intensive Care, heart trouble and only able to see Bunny. I felt so guilty for going. I had no idea how major an op she was having but Mum being Mum, she hadn't wanted to worry me and put my feelings first as usual. But the scars healed, the tubes and stitches came out, and a couple of weeks later, I was walking Mum up and down outside in the August sunshine.

I have some strange memories of that time. I remember speeding back from the Woodland Hospital with my brother, going way too fast, having borrowed Bunny's car. I prepared a meal for Mum, to feed her through the PEG she had in her stomach. Months later I think she was embarrassed by the memory as no one apart from Bunny had done this before. But hey, I thought, this is the woman who changed my nappies; so a little liquid lunch is no problem. Mum is still the same loving, caring, person she always was. She takes a bit longer with her food and has even more cream on her dessert than I do, but she's the same person.

I also remember the radiotherapy mask pretty vividly; this strange, clear head-shaped mask with arrows and squiggles on it, and holes for where it screwed down. She's a lot braver than me – I'd have run a mile.

I haven't thought about the details of what happened that summer for a long time and bits keep coming back to me as I've been making a list for this piece. Another strange memory fragment is when some of us watched an old family video. It looked like Christmas from a few years ago with children coming and going. This voice kept coming in from off-screen, and Mum asked who it was. "It's you, don't you recognise yourself?" we asked her.

I met my future wife that summer and I remember not wanting to tire Mum until she was better as she was still recovering. But how proud I was to introduce Vanessa to her when I brought her home for the first time. Vanessa is expecting our third child as I write and if all goes well Mum will have seven grandchildren by February 2007, six of whom she'd never have seen but for the surgery.

Meeting more of the people from FACEFAX at the weekend (my in-laws have just hosted an event to raise money for Mum's support group) and hearing their stories, I realise how lucky we all are. Another family friend died from a similar tumour and we were so lucky that Mum came through. She is one of the lucky ones and eight years on, we're on borrowed time as a family.

This story has a happy ending with Mum and Bunny marrying up in Orkney the year after her op and the whole family gathering round. James back from Australia; Vanessa and I engaged; and Clare and Connor, all together as a family.

Carol takes up the story

LOOKING back, there was a clear and defining moment when I knew that my life was about to change forever.

I had been working for nearly ten years at a local ceramics company as head of their decorating department, where I oversaw six girls whom I taught and trained in ceramic skills. We were a very happy team despite the heat, the stifling airlessness, the noise and fumes from the six huge kilns and the ever-pervading dust from the baked ceramic clay. And of course, the constantly stressful and pressured working environment.

As time progressed, I became increasingly involved in the design aspect of the company. This entailed visits to London, where we worked with many major stores such as Harrods, Selfridges, Liberty, Conran and John Lewis. We also designed for the Fauve Exhibition at The Royal Academy and The National Gallery as well as frequently working with such famous people as Marco Pierre White, Gordon Ramsay and Cameron Mackintosh. I regularly travelled to the Stoke on Trent potteries where we had a large factory and I met with buyers and designers while still overseeing the decorating department back in Northampton. Life was hectic and fun and I loved the involvement with creativity. This was a major part of my life.

By 1998 I had become even more caught up in the frenetic whirlpool at work when one day my boss Jim Powell suggested that I fly to Tokyo for three weeks to meet important Japanese clients for whom I had been designing various items of tableware.

I was to be invited as their guest. It was a tremendous honour and I was to go as 'the famous Carol Kimbell, designer from Northampton'. But the actual emotions I felt were utter horror and shock.

Perhaps it was fear of the unknown. Or my fear of flying. Or the fact that I was going to make the trip alone. But I was absolutely petrified. I sensed that somehow I had reached a crossroads in my life; that somehow my fate was already sealed and that my life would be changed forever. Now I often wonder if that shock triggered something else within my body.

I was becoming very tired and run down, which I initially put down to work-overload, stress and a very busy and fully committed family life. I had lost weight, my hair was getting very thin and I was very breathless. This was diagnosed by my GP as arterial fibrillation. But I had also developed an ulcer on the back of my tongue, which just would not heal despite several courses of antibiotics. However, I continued with my preparations as my state of health seemed of little importance compared with the adventure that awaited me in Japan.

Tokyo was hugely exciting for me, flying with Japan Airlines, staying in a Japanese hotel, being looked after by my own personal guide, Yuko, and having two personal interpreters. I was kept very busy: painting, giving demonstrations, having business meetings and being entertained, without any letup.

Japan also presented a huge culture shock with its many millions of people, high-rise buildings, noise, earth tremors and above all, overpowering humidity. I felt unwell with earache, a sore jaw and an ulcerated mouth. Everything seemed oppressive, perhaps because I was feeling so unwell. I thought to myself that as soon as I got back home I would get this sorted out, little realising just how ill I really was. But this was the experience of a lifetime and I was not going to let some silly sore throat ruin my trip.

After getting home, I made an appointment at my GP's surgery and saw Catherine Blackman. She listened carefully to my account of symptoms, examined me and, rather to my surprise, recommended a second opinion and made an appointment with the ENT specialist at Northampton General Hospital. The specialist was away and as Catherine felt the delay would be too long she made another appointment for me to see Mr Clive Pratt, the Maxillofacial Consultant, based at Woodlands Hospital in Kettering. This was a private appointment so I was to see him in a matter of days.

Although elated to be home, I also felt exhausted and generally unfit. My hair was terribly thin and I had lost more weight, but none of this rang alarm bells with me. I was relieved that at last something was happening.

It was a painful examination and the consultation included an x-ray of the jaw and neck area. Mr Pratt told me not to worry and confidently added, "We can sort this out."

I was admitted for a minor operation, which actually turned out to be three hours in duration and included a biopsy. I felt particularly in the dark at this stage and the word 'cancer' had not been mentioned. Following the operation I had a bad morphine reaction and felt very unwell and very sick. I still heard no alarm bells ringing but there were tiny niggles of doubt which were beginning to worry me. I was allowed home and told to await the result of the biopsy.

The results were back in days and I was given an appointment to see Mr Pratt for the results. Bunny, my partner, came with me, both of us feeling rather nervous and unsure. I remember wearing a dark blue jacket and skirt, feeling confident in my appearance and wanting to create a positive impression.

Bunny and I had to wait for what seemed an age before we were finally called in. Upon entering the room I was aware of many other people standing at the back, in what seemed to be a line. Mr Pratt came forward and asked us both to sit down. Bunny was on one side of the room while I was placed in an examination chair. This made me feel very isolated from Bunny and butterflies churned about in my stomach.

Everyone looked so serious and they were very quiet. Mr Pratt spoke gently to me: "I am very sorry." But what followed I can barely remember, except that it was a grade three tumour and they could, he assured me, do something about it.

He was pretty certain that it was 'the primary site' but he added that it would have to be a 'belt and braces job' and I remember thinking, "What on earth does that mean?"

Everything was then explained very carefully. 'Belt and braces' meant surgery to remove the tumour, followed by radiotherapy. Bunny seemed miles apart from me and all I wanted was to be with him. We hardly dared look at each other. I desperately needed reassurance and I remember looking at everyone standing in the room, which felt heavily charged with concern.

Dr Macmillan, a very kindly man, introduced himself as my consultant radiotherapist and said he would be looking after me later on. He asked if he might look in my mouth. In my confusion, I thought he was connected to the Macmillan Nurses or Hospice, little realising that this just happened to be his name!

Other people spoke, but I don't remember what they said. I do recall asking Mr Pratt what the operation meant and he said, almost apologetically that it could last up to 12 hours. This was another shock and I wondered if my heart would stand up to it.

"How important is this surgery?" I asked nervously. "Very important. There can be no other decision," he replied. I was definitely to have surgery and radiotherapy. There was no question of one without the other.

Mr Pratt told me the way to approach this was to be very positive. He knew from experience that there were two choices; either turn my face to the wall (i.e. give up) or turn away from the wall and fight. I have never forgotten these words and how true they are. Somehow, somewhere, in the days, weeks and months to follow, I summoned every ounce of strength to fight back. This was not going to beat me. But at that moment, sitting in the consulting room and feeling like a complete stranger to myself, I did not feel confident.

Most of what then happened is now a blurred image; the memory of us walking back to the car park, feeling completely dazed, the whole world tipped over, and all that was familiar now sharply in focus, huge and surreal. How on earth was I going to break this news to my family and what would happen to us all now?

Bunny was a rock and became, thank God, very practical, which helped make the world shift back into a position I could almost recognise. But how scared we both were! The unknown had become the known and beyond that, who knew what lay ahead?

So much happened between that day of reckoning and my admittance to Kettering General Hospital for what I call the big op. There were endless check-ups with Mr Pratt and his staff and I had an MRI scan, alien and daunting, but so terribly necessary. I had to lie for an age inside a long tube, not daring to move as much as an eye muscle while loud banging and clunking noises went on as the machine did its clever work. Fortunately I didn't have to do it again as by then I had virtually frozen into a corpse.

I then had a feeding tube known as a 'PEG' inserted into my stomach. This was a most uncomfortable procedure that takes place under local anaesthetic. It was an absolute necessity and literally proved a lifesaver in the months to come, especially after my radiation treatment. I learnt to live with 'Billy', as I called it, for nine months. And though I was glad when the time came for him to go, I felt somewhat vulnerable for a while without him.

Much information about mouth cancer, or cancer of the soft tissue, was gleaned on the Internet while I took every opportunity to ask medical friends pertinent and relevant questions. Barry Nuttall, our friend and family doctor was by now back from his holiday, aghast to hear the news. He immediately called in, calmed us all down and gave us wise and valuable advice. He is a philosophical man and this was much appreciated. Indeed, his presence was never far away from then on, and he is still keeping a watchful eye on me all these years later. It is good to have a doctor in the house.

I also bombarded Mr Pratt, as I needed to know all the answers. This was MY BODY, MY LIFE, which we were discussing and I had to take some charge at this stage.

Shockingly, I learned that I would have my front lower jaw broken in two, to gain access to the tumour at the back of my tongue in the tonsil area. Then my lower face would be opened up, rather like the pages of a book. I would also have lymph glands removed from my neck and horror of horrors (vanity coming to the fore) I might lose some of my teeth.

I would also lose one third of my tongue and have a large flap of skin/tissue/muscle/veins, (called a 'free flap') taken from my lower left arm (I'm right handed.) This would be removed by another surgeon and inserted precisely into the area from which the tumour had been removed. In other words, they would rebuild my throat with my arm. To replace the surgical wound on my arm, another skin graft was to be taken from my forearm.

Fortunately, I don't have very hairy arms, but much later I would meet other fellow patients who would joke with some hilarity about their tickly, hairy throats. I understand that this does not last forever, thank heavens.

There was more to come, some of which affected a large area of muscle in the shoulder area. I realised that my left arm/shoulder/neck area would probably be out of action for a while. In my case this required considerable physiotherapy at the hospital for several months and happily improved the situation significantly.

I was also warned of the possibility of my jawbone being affected by more cancerous cells. If this was discovered, bone would be removed from my thighbone and grafted into a 'new jawbone.' So, apparently, my body parts had many uses welded into new places here and there. "Terrific," I told myself, "This is not an option." Skin grafts could also be problematic. Sometimes they would reject themselves and new areas would have to be found, possibly high in the front chest area or at the side of the temple area. Luckily my skin grafts and transplants worked and healed quite rapidly.

Armed with all this information and realising that the op was a lifesaver, I still asked, or rather tried to insist that Mr Pratt would please, please try his hardest to save my teeth. I recall him smiling. And yes, he did. He was brilliant.

During the build-up to my op, I must admit I was scared and I realised that I looked unwell. The time lapse must have been about three weeks and I had much to do tidying up all my personal affairs and spending precious time with my family and visitors. I was getting tired. I did wonder if I would get through all of this and many times my confidence plummeted to zero.

Then a miracle occurred. Some very dear friends suggested that I see a hypnotherapist, someone they already knew and who was tried and trusted. The visit was quite remarkable. He was the very same anaesthetist who had been present at my first operation and biopsy and I immediately knew that he could help.

During several visits he talked me through my fears, at the same time recording a tape to take into hospital with me. I found this invaluable and played the tape on the eve and dawn of my surgery, as well as all the way down to the theatre and it had a most calming effect.

Throughout this time I was in a state of limbo. For this was the dawn of realisation. I had cancer and was going into hospital for major surgery, which 'please God' was going to keep me alive. My family and friends were unbelievably understanding and good to me and without their support I'm certain I would not be here today. I know I am an incredibly fortunate human being to have them all around me, even now. It makes me feel so humble and I thank them all from the bottom of my heart.

I also know that without the incredible skill, understanding and kindness from Mr Pratt and the theatre and ward staff, intensive care unit, oncology staff, speech therapist, physiotherapists and of course Barry, I would not have survived. I know many others were receiving care from these dedicated people too but this all seemed so personal to me.

The momentous day finally arrived. I was admitted the night before the big op into a small room opposite the nurses' station in A. M. Lee Ward at Kettering General Hospital. Many different members of staff came to check me out, introducing themselves as part of the team. Bunny and my sisters Inga and Judy were with me, giving all their strength and support. I had already said my farewells to my children, Alastair, Clare and James and we all joked about the dawn of a new 'me', a new Mummy, who would have an amazing face-lift and no more saggy chins.

Alastair, my eldest son, was by now winging his way across the world to spend time in Australia and I wished him well. It was hard saying goodbye, but being positive for us both, I assured him that all would be just fine. James, my younger son, having newly graduated, was at home. He was also planning a year trip to Australia, hoping to meet up with his brother. James could not leave until later and would wait until the operation was over and I had started my radiotherapy. Clare, my daughter and her young son, Connor, my first grandchild, lived nearby, constantly giving support, love and laughter. They would be seeing me after the surgery.

Mr Pratt arrived later that evening and while talking to us all, produced a pen and began making marks, lines and dots on my left arm, jokingly referring to this as a fine work of art. I realised this was to indicate the area for the skin flap or graft. A considerate nurse then asked if we would like to see the intensive care unit where I would recover from the op.

Apparently it would be two days before I would be brought back gently into a state of consciousness. I felt the need to see where I would lose these days and I knew that we all felt reassured on making this visit. Later that night, while on my own, I wrote letters to Bunny, my children and my two sisters. This was important.

Dawn arrived all too soon and a feeling of unreality took over. It was an empty feeling. Bunny arrived and stayed with me all the way to the operating theatre, smiling, talking, holding my hand. Heaven knows what he must have been going through. My family were my rock, supporting and loving me throughout my illness, giving me a strong sense of survival. They needed me as much as I needed them. My life was in the hands of my surgeon and his wonderful team. My Guardian Angel was there and I gave myself to them all with trust and hope.

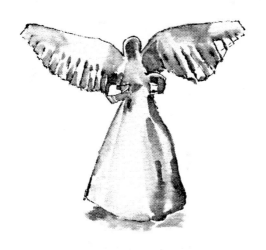

Bunny makes the first of many journeys

WAITING for news is difficult. One's imagination makes great leaps in just about every direction possible. There are no facts available, just feelings and fears.

I remember the drive Carol and I took to see the surgeon, Mr Pratt, who had the results of the biopsy. It was a beautiful sunny day. The journey was about 14 miles, enough time for both of us to hold hands and persuade each other that we would shortly return home with Good News.

Deep down, I think we both of us knew that I would be making this journey again many times – but next time the sun would not be my companion.

On arrival we were called in and holding hands we entered a large rectangular, sunny room. I have little memory of further events after the hammer-blow news that Carol had cancer. I was looking at Carol all the time – she was the only focus of my attention, apart from hearing the disconnected phrases of 'belt and braces' and 'we are confident' but nothing more. In fact nothing more at all, not even the journey home. Shock does amazing things to our memory recall at times.

What a deep sea we now all lived in – plenty of optimistic light on the surface, thank God, but very dark in the depths of those private moments. Then things began to move very fast. In a sense, the blur of so many events was a blessing for there was so much to do so quickly.

It was another sunny day when we drove to hospital for Carol's admission. Not much was said, but once again there was a lot of holding of hands. That kind of touching didn't need many words.

The staff was kind and understanding, calm and attentive. I could see a tear in Carol's eyes. The nurses could not, but I knew those eyes too well. However, there is a sort of mechanical inevitability involved with the preparation for a major operation. Many tests, many questions, many marks being made on arms and neck and worst of all, many forms being completed and signed.

Early next morning I accompanied Carol to the anaesthetist's room, holding hands all the way, even when they administered those drugs, which would take her away from me. I told Carol that I loved her and slowly, while looking at me all the time and smiling, she drifted into unconsciousness. I was then very gently asked to leave the room. The thoughts that were going through my head – or perhaps I was even saying them out loud, I don't know – were that she should find strength through my strength in some spiritual way and that the surgeons could completely release her from the cancer and not find that it had already spread to other areas in her body. I drove back to work. It was a long, long day.

I received news late in the evening that Carol was out of theatre and now in Intensive Care. The message also tried to 'reassure' me that she was 'comfortable'. I made some important calls and headed for the hospital. Upon arrival, the staff guided me to a small room near the Intensive Care Unit, obviously for next of kin to stay close to their loved ones. This room must have witnessed a thousand emotions before mine and I waited and waited for news.

It seemed like hours but suddenly a nurse appeared and said I could see Carol briefly. She explained that Carol was still unconscious and that I had to be prepared for the shock of her appearance – apparently quite normal for this type of operation.

I followed her into Intensive Care and was taken to the far bed where two nurses were attending Carol. I had to stand away from the bed to allow them constant access to the equipment surrounding her. She was literally wired and plugged in. There was buzzing, beeping, flashing and pumping with every life-saving device operating at once. I felt both reassured and yet frightened for Carol. I wasn't allowed to touch her but I was asked to talk to her. Apparently the hearing is the first sense that returns after trauma but there was no response. I was assured that this did not mean she hadn't heard me and then I was asked to leave. But I was grateful to the staff for letting me see Carol so soon after the operation.

After two days, Carol regained consciousness and was moved back to the ward. I was relieved and thought that this was real progress but it didn't last. Carol unfortunately relapsed and this time it was her heart which was giving concern to the doctors. Ironically, her progress from the actual operation was going well but the intense strain of physical trauma and constant coughing had brought on another potentially more dangerous condition.

Carol being taken back into Intensive Care was traumatic for us all and we redoubled our efforts to try and tell her that everything was getting better and that she seemed to be responding well to the new treatments. We all hoped that this was the case.

I don't remember which visit it was when I 'popped the question', but we were on our own, holding hands again and I just said, "Will you marry me?"

We looked at each other, she smiled and immediately mouthed "Yes, yes." What great joy. A surge of excitement went through both of us. Don't ask me how, but we both knew then that she was going to get better and fast.

Carol tells of her terrible isolation

THERE was a flash of light, tunnel vision, voices, faces and Clare, my daughter with someone else beside her looming into my vision. She was speaking to me: "Mummy." And then she was gone and there was darkness. I can only liken this experience to a television being turned on, with its sound and light and images and just as abruptly, turned off again.

Unknown to me, Clare, James and Bunny were all there beside the recovery bed. But the next time I came out of my dark, deep sleep I was very awake. I was lying on a bed, somewhere in a room. Strange noises behind me were coming from the machinery I was connected up to and two people were moving about near me. I looked for the nursery murals on the walls. I had been told to expect to see them on regaining consciousness after two days of oblivion. But there were only blank walls with nothing there. "I'm dead. I must be dead," I thought.

Then I was sick and I realized I was very much alive. The next biggest impact was that I was completely immobilised. I was attached to all sorts of machinery, I had a tracheostomy and my left arm was heavily bandaged. I was aware of a terrible feeling of isolation. I wasn't in pain, but I was unable to speak. Whatever I was wired up to was doing its essential work but there was no communication until the nurses administered to me. At some point I must have been delivered back to A. M. Lee Ward, where I was greeted with such kindness.

That night I had an additional complication and was aware that I had a nurse beside me at all times. Her name was Eileen. I was still connected up to various pieces of machinery, churning away and I began to feel extremely unwell. I had a very heavy chest pain and was struggling for breath through the ghastly tracheostomy. I knew this wasn't right and judging by the alarm and consternation on Eileen's face, it dawned upon me that this situation could no longer continue.

Of course, I couldn't speak and whenever I was asked a question I could communicate only with my eyes. Then Mr Pratt arrived and the next thing I knew I was being whisked back to Intensive Care. I felt utterly despondent; what on earth was happening to me now? All my strength and resolve vanished. I can barely remember what happened after that but I knew I was very ill. I couldn't understand why but I also knew I was in the best possible place if I was going to recover from this.

Intensive Care affected me quite deeply. The dedication and caring is unbelievable and I was not left alone for a moment. Time lapsed into unreality again and perhaps I was hallucinating. I certainly had terrible nightmares. I couldn't move at all and the tracheostomy, my lifeline, was still attached to me. I had a very painful left arm but I don't remember any other pain – just a tiredness I cannot describe. It was like falling into a big black hole forever and ever, with no desire or effort to climb back out. Looking back, I realize I was giving up. A very special nurse sat with me all night, holding my hand and this meant so much to me. Human, physical contact is so vital and I really believe touch has healing power. Machinery can seem so deadly and unresponsive and I desperately needed a smile, a touch, reassurance and comfort.

Gradually I began to be aware that sometimes Bunny was there too, holding my right hand, smiling and talking to me. But I felt so tired.

Something else happened. I have thought very carefully as to whether or not I should share this part of my journey but I think it is important that I should because it was such a special experience for me. My sisters and I had discussed before the op that we should have a 'place' where we could meet in spirit during the time of surgery and recovery. We decided upon a beautiful beach on the Isle of Sanday in the Orkneys.

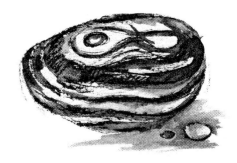

Orkney is special. It is where my childhood holidays were spent and where my mother and her parents came from. It is where I continue to return every year and maintain contact with all my close cousins who live there. Bunny and I now have a small place there, which we love. It is my touchstone for solace, my spiritual home.

I became aware of 'floating' as if I was being gently carried along. I had arrived at the beach on Sunday and I stood in the dunes looking for my sisters. I couldn't see them and I tried and tried to get down onto the beach, but couldn't. At last I felt at peace, the tiredness and fatigue dissipating.

Then a miracle occurred. Bunny was at my side, back in the Intensive Care Unit, and he asked me to marry him. I couldn't speak, but I was so overjoyed that all I could do was mouth, "YES, YES".

The next thing was a letter, which Bunny read aloud to me. It was from Claire O-J, my dearest friend. She said, "Fight . . . don't give up" and much later when we discussed the timing of this letter, she told me she had been driven by some strong force to write immediately. I still have that letter to this day.

I began to regain some strength and at last realised that in order to attract attention, I could knock the 'clip' off my toe or finger, wherever it happened to be attached. This would immediately set off an alarm and help would be at hand. Feeling so vulnerable, I was utterly and completely in the hands of this wonderful, caring team.

One day a nurse asked me if I would like to hear some music and I silently nodded. He had brought his radio in and tuned it into Classic FM. The purity of that sound was like a gift from heaven after all the horrors of before. I must have been improving because I was longing to see daylight and the sky, hear the birds singing, the sound of the wind and rain – contact with the outside world.

Medical staff came and went, assessing my progress and at last I heard, joy of joys, the words: "She can go back to A. M. Lee Ward." I had been in Intensive Care for six days.

Bunny sees Carol
make progress

SOMETIMES you wonder just how much progress can be made in a few days. Carol was now back in control. She was able to cope with visitors beyond the immediate family and making very sure that her appearance was as presentable as possible.

When you see vanity rear its head again, you know that the lady is getting back into action. It wasn't long before Carol's thoughts turned to leaving hospital and returning home to some sort of normality.

Inga recalls her
tokens of love

"YES, its cancer" was the phone call I had been dreading and here was my sister over 300 miles away, bravely giving me the results of her biopsy. All I wanted to do was go south to be with her, but my children were both still young and at school so it was not possible.

So then began a whole new era. We kept in touch daily and I would send a small package as often as possible containing books, charms, crystals and other things I have long since forgotten. A dear friend of mine, who is currently being treated for Leukaemia, commented on the kindness of friends and all the gifts they had brought her. Is this some basic instinct to nurture the sick? We would love to give the gift of healing but it is not within our power, so we give tokens instead.

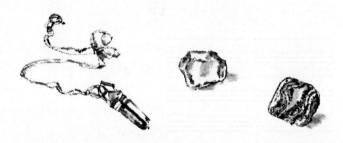

A whole new vocabulary now entered our everyday speech; tumours, MRI scan, radiotherapy, masks, feeding tube, and grafts. The details of Carol's treatment sounded terrifying. In order to remove the tumour at the back of her tongue, the surgeons were going to have to cut through her jaw, and after the removal of the tumour, her throat was to be reconstructed with skin grafts from her arm. More terrifying still was the possibility that her face might be paralysed and her speech lost, not to mention her sense of taste and a few teeth into the bargain. Carol's teeth were very important to her and she still has them to this day so the surgeon must have been extremely skilled to be able to preserve them.

Eventually a date was set for Carol's operation and I travelled south overnight with a friend to be with Carol, her family and our sister, Judy. I remember arriving at Judy's house, which had been our old family home and the reality of what lay ahead was overwhelming. I confess I could easily have driven away with my friend, pretending that nothing was happening.

And then to see Carol. The next few days passed in a haze of activity and visits from her family and friends. I remember us going arm in arm to a fete in the village and people greeting Carol and wishing her well. It was almost a carnival atmosphere.

And then to see Carol's surgeon the night before her operation – the cancer was calling the shots again. Mr Pratt explained the procedure for the following day, and I remember him drawing lines on her arm to show where the skin graft would come from. We were also shown the Intensive Care Unit where Carol would be taken after the operation, a long room with a line of beds facing the nurses' station and two side rooms at each end with windows looking onto the ward. One of the side rooms was painted with animals, and I remember Mr Pratt joking that if Carol came round in this room, she was not to think she was in the jungle!

And then of course we had to leave her, and I don't remember any of us shedding a tear. The time for tears had passed. Carol had told me she had brought her make-up with her and was planning to put on make-up for the operation, so that was the strange thought I went away with.

I stayed in Carol's house on the day of the operation to feel closer to her. Bunny, Judy and Clare were there also and it rained and indeed thundered that day. It was a very long day and seemed an eternity before Bunny was eventually given the news that the operation was over, and that Carol was stable and in intensive care.

The next day Bunny was told he could visit Carol again but he was to be the only one. I decided to go with him in any case and was allowed into the Intensive Care Unit as well. While the nurse was explaining to us what to expect, I began to look around and saw someone lying very peacefully to my right. Then slowly I realised it was Carol. She looked so peaceful and there was no sign of her scar. Her skin was pure and her hair was pushed back from her face. She looked like a child again and not the battle veteran I had been preparing myself to see and I cannot tell you how relieved I felt.

Of course there were many more fights to come. Learning to talk again, learning to eat again (it is surprising just what Carol is able to eat now) and of course the radiotherapy treatment. But the worst was over. When at last Carol was able to leave hospital, she went to recuperate with her mother-in-law Peggy. She has the most wonderful organic vegetable garden and she made many delicious pureed vegetable dishes for Carol, which I am sure, must have aided her recovery.

Carol and I had been planning a holiday in Spain to stay with one of our cousins before her cancer was diagnosed. Heulyn has the most beautiful house set in the mountains above Malaga, built in an olive grove and called Al Munia meaning 'The Garden'. I decided to go there anyway after the nightmare operation was over and found some peace. Indeed, I am writing this in Al Munia and Carol and Bunny are here as well. It is our third visit and we continue to find peace here.

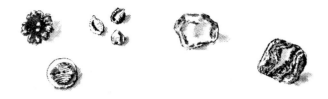

Judy discovers a way
to communicate

WHEN Carol broke the news to me that she had cancer, despite the fact that deep down inside I had prepared myself to face that fact, I was still absolutely shocked to the core. My sister had cancer. That is the most horrifying beast to confront. I knew though, that I had to lock horns with this demon. I could and would not walk out of this nightmare for my sister's sake – we were in this together and the fight was on.

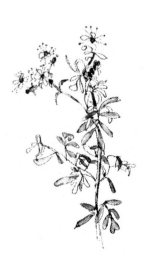

I was filled with a dreadful foreboding but knew I had to be positive and brave for Carol, give her my strength and fight back hard, despite the emotional turmoil we were all going through. We decided to look on this cancer 'thing' as a challenge, taking one day at a time and being open about it. So we paced

29

and talked and hugged and howled. Carol was inspirational and brave and I think I drew my strength from her just as much as she did from me. I could not and would not let her down. I was there for her no matter what this beast could throw at us.

The days leading up to her operation passed slowly, every hurdle was confronted and come to terms with. Any information – and there was plenty – was readily dissected and absorbed. We realised there would be changes, real life challenging changes. But through all of this there was hope as well as we clung miserably to the wreckage of ourselves on a very stormy sea.

We were told that Carol might not be able to speak again. Or if she did, it would be very different as her speech would be altered profoundly due to the radical nature of the surgery. This was very hard to comprehend and come to terms with but daily we became better at dealing with our emotions. We were coping – but only just.

We discussed how she would feel after the op, and what she wanted from us. We knew that the five senses, especially smell and touch would become very important to Carol. It was agreed I would bring in sweet smelling herbs and flowers for her to smell and that I would give light massages to her feet, legs and hands. I made up a box of talismans for Carol to have: bits of stone and wood from Orkney, a silver sixpence, pebbles, beads and love tokens – anything that held power and was meaningful to Carol. We devised a special place where we could all go to in our thoughts, a beautiful beach on Sanday in the Orkney Islands, which we had found and loved that summer. We could all go there mentally and meet; it was a way of sharing, of reaching out and of being together while being apart.

Seeing Carol in Intensive Care after her 12-hour operation was the scariest thing. I felt panicky, helpless and backed up against a wall. All my instincts screamed for me to flee. As she had a tracheostomy and could not speak, I devised a 'Point Card'. This listed all the main words she needed to describe how she was or what she wanted. So all she had to do was point at the permutation of words she needed to make us understand. It gave her a silent 'voice' and I felt better for doing something useful and for keeping her occupied during this anxious time.

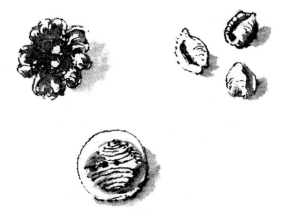

Carol gradually improved and regained her strength and sense of humour. She came out of ITU and into her own room. And one day when I went to visit, a miracle happened – she actually spoke to me.

With great effort and satisfaction she said, "I'm back!" She most certainly was

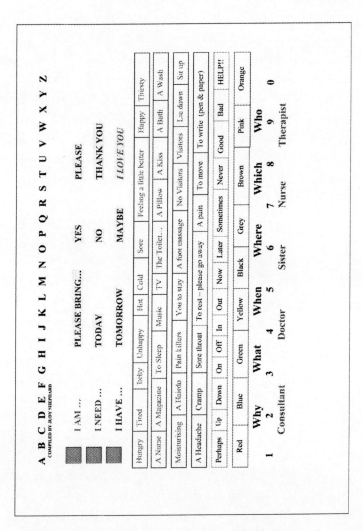

The Point Card, devised by Judy Shephard

Carol comes out of
Intensive Care

ARRIVING back at A. M. Lee Ward was such a mixture of emotions. The nurses were overjoyed to get me back again in their care as my traumatic departure for Intensive Care had left them full of concern and dismay. Now I was back and my room was overflowing with flowers and cards. I burst into tears, which is not very easy when you have a tube stuck in your throat. I must have gurgled quite a lot.

The relief was enormous. I was alive and I just knew with such a powerful certainty I would get better. I could see my family again and there would be a future. I still had a long way to go but I knew I could do it.

Then began a routine, which was comforting in its very predictability. My surgeon Mr Pratt was there every day and there were numerous visits from physiotherapists, dieticians, staff from the Haematology and Pathology Departments and my speech therapist, Brent Gibbons and many others. Dr Baines my heart specialist and Mr Bill Smith, who is now my present Maxillofacial consultant, also came. He had operated on me with Mr Pratt and Mr Smith still looks after me all these years later, patiently listening to my accounts of well-being, as well as my ups and downs.

After a few days the tracheostomy was removed and that same day my sister Judy was allowed to visit me. It was her first visit to the ward since all the previous dramas and I had discovered that by pressing my finger to the area where the 'stoma' was, I could make a noise. Much to her surprise and delight, I managed to utter, "I'm back." We were euphoric and we wept.

My immediate, close family were allowed to visit me and they worked so hard to encourage and support me. My other sister Inga was still away in Spain, but my son Alastair had come home from Australia. Most of my family were now around me and I was thrilled to see them all.

Every day I received more flowers, cards and letters from my large family and friends and from people I didn't even know. I was utterly dumbstruck, quite literally, by all the kindness, caring and love – what healing power.

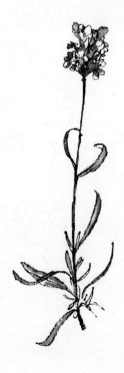

Some of my memories have faded, but I have also found there is almost too much to say and therefore I have picked out just a few important memories.

I was unable to turn over without assistance and a wonderful night sister of 'the old school' plumped up my pillows in just the right place for my aching back so I slept like a baby.

There was my first stumble out of the room, helped by two nurses, to the bathroom. We made it and at last I had a bath, albeit on a kind of slide or plank. And after washing my hair I began to feel human again.

Later there was my friend Joy, blow-drying my hair for me,

setting me to rights and making me laugh. That meant so much to me. Scatters No. 2, as Joy is fondly known in our family, had cancer many years ago. She was and is a survivor. I'm Scatters No. 1 because I'm older then her.

Judy came in with a huge bunch of freshly picked herbs from her garden and mine. The scent of herbs can, even now, transport me right back to that time. It's so evocative. And the massages she gave my poor feet . . . what bliss.

Also Jane, my other 'sister' and my best friend, managed to sneak in at a time when only immediate family were allowed to visit. She appeared quite unexpectedly by my bedside and she didn't falter for a moment when she saw my frightening face. I could have hugged her and when she left I felt so much better.

Then there was Alastair, walking with me up and down the ward and always encouraging me. And once I began to gain more strength, just pushing me to do that little bit more.

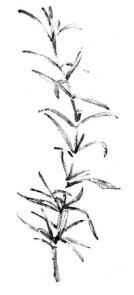

Inga phoned me from Spain, delighted to hear my funny, strange voice. It was hardly a voice really, but I was there and could say, "Hello." Inga would be coming to see me on her return from Spain, en route home to Edinburgh.

Clare and James came in with relief on their faces. At last 'Mum' was back and life had some normality again.

And, of course Bunny was there every day, driving miles to

and from Kettering. His visits were more than often twice a day and I eagerly looked forward to them. He would bring news from friends and tell me what was happening in the village, at home, at work, constantly keeping me in touch with the world outside the hospital.

One day, I summoned up the courage to look in a mirror. It had already been explained to me that I might feel more reassured if I had someone there with me and not to do it on my own. But I'm stubborn and I did it on my own. I remember quite distinctly that I looked shocking. I was almost recognisable but was that really me or was it someone else staring back?

I had many stitches on my face, right around my neck and up behind my ear. But the main shock was my swollen face, due to fluid building up because my lymph glands had been removed and the fluid had nowhere to drain to. I looked like a zombie or something out of a horror film. "Horrendous," I thought – but much to my amazement, once the stitches had all been removed from my face and neck, I began to visibly improve.

I was told I had two metal plates and pins in my jawbone to hold the broken bone together but it certainly didn't seem to cause any pain. My left arm was still bandaged and very swollen, leaving me with a useless left hand.

Every now and then it would be unbandaged, reassessed and perhaps a few more stitches would be removed. My arm still hurt like hell, in spite of painkillers, but I knew it would improve in time. My right arm was not much better, due to all the injections I had in Intensive Care. Most injections were now going into my stomach or bottom. It's amazing what you can get used to.

Another interesting fact was that apparently I no longer had a pulse in my left wrist. What a macabre thought. Now I can laugh about it, but in fact, although I joke now, if I were to be found somewhere with only my left arm sticking out, I would be pronounced dead. It's not really such a funny thought after all. Perhaps I should wear a bracelet with the relevant information engraved on it. And this is an interesting predicament that must apply to many other fellow patients.

I did worry about my impaired speech and difficulty swallowing. Brent Gibbons, my ever-patient speech therapist, showed me how to form certain syllables with my maimed tongue and I would practise. But it was hard. He also persuaded me to try swallowing yoghurt and to try drinking water. This would result in getting drenched, with water all over the bed. I just couldn't do it, not even with a straw.

I actually found it easier to manage a thicker fluid like milk because somehow it would slip down without my spluttering and choking like an old asthmatic cat. Food was a problem. I still had Billy the food PEG, so obviously there was no chance of starving to death. But I was losing a lot of weight, which is perhaps understandable for any of us in these circumstances. *(Readers trying to lose weight are advised 'not to try this at home.')*

Sometimes lunch or supper would arrive and all I could do was bleakly stare at it. If it wasn't liquidized up into some form of gooey mush, like baby food, it was fairly impossible to swallow. There is a small section in this book with helpful tips, which hopefully might be of some use at this stage.

But remember, this was back in 1998 and awareness of such difficulties has now much improved.

The other very important happening was the Point Card that Judy devised. This was a lifesaver and apart from allowing me to communicate with everyone, it also caused much amusement. A slightly more polite version is now used in various hospitals and it would be rewarding to think it could be used on a much wider scale for many patients have difficulty in speech communication.

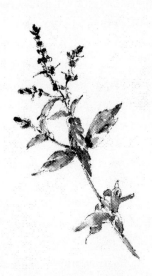

Finally, the day came when I was allowed to go home. Bunny collected me and it had been agreed by all the family that I should stay at first with Peggy, my mother-in-law. This was a wonderful respite for me. It was another healing time and calmness and order took place together with love and kindness. I was back home in familiar surroundings in the village I had been brought up in.

Every day I grew stronger. I was still having regular checkups and visits from the nurse and I needed help to bathe, as I wasn't strong enough to manage this on my own. Very gradually I would walk around the garden, a bit farther every day, but always with some help. I had visitors, my family and friends – not too many yet – but I was overjoyed to see them all.

Best of all was the wonderful food Peggy would prepare for me, fresh from the vegetable garden; always pureed so I could swallow it down and full of goodness. I'm convinced this helped my rapidly increasing recovery. It might have taken hours for me to eat it all, but most importantly, I was beginning to enjoy my food again despite all the surgery that had taken place.

My speech, though impaired, was also manageable. The scars on my face and neck were already fading a lot with a bit of help from Vitamin E ointments and an eye ointment prescribed by the Hospital. I had to exercise my hands with soft rubber balls as they were still swollen and needed to regain strength. Apparently my thumb and index fingers would always remain quite numb due to the surgery that had taken place on my arm.

Eight years later, my hand has much improved but it will probably never be 100 per cent and I do tend to drop things quite easily. But at least I have the use back to a degree of acceptable normality.

One of the worst problems for me was the amount of fluid, saliva, which would build up in my mouth, causing quite a few difficulties with my speech. I hated this and unfortunately no one could tell me if this would improve. I also knew I still had the radiotherapy to come.

However, for that period of time while staying with Peggy and her family, I was finding myself again. I was even managing to concentrate enough to read a little and write a few letters and I was happy to be moving forwards.

Then one day I was back home again in my own house. It was summer and our wonderful friend Roger Wilkin (Bunny's childhood friend) had been busy tidying up the garden for my homecoming. Margaret, my long time help who has rallied round through thick and thin, had been beavering away in the house and everything, everywhere, looked fantastic.

I had such a welcome home from everyone, including two very boisterous and over-excited dogs, Robin and Amy. Overwhelmed, I found the whole homecoming experience almost too much to comprehend. But when all the excitement had died down, my lovely cousin, Elsa, phoned to say she was coming over from Oxford to see me. Unbeknown to me, Jane (my 'other sister') and Judy had obtained a wheel chair from somewhere and Elsa, Jane and Judy were all going to take me out on a little trip.

Elsa appeared, her arms laden with various assorted, brightly coloured scarves, small and large, soft, silky and floaty. Some of these had belonged to her mother, my Aunty Helen and I was delighted to receive them. My neck was still quite noticeably scarred from the surgery and I knew I would need them during and after radiotherapy.

I was duly packed into a car, alongside the wheelchair, and off we drove to Althorp House and gardens. This was my first outing and I loved every minute of it. I was just pushed and pulled around the beautiful gardens, down to the lake where Princess Di had been buried, finally ending up in the café area. What to others must have seemed quite a normal day out was such a day of laughter and happiness for me.

There was another appointment to see Mr Pratt and he seemed pleased with my progress. Everything in my mouth was healing well and the scars on my neck and chin, although still red, were definitely improving. My arm was still a problem. Most of the stitches had been removed but the wound wasn't healing as fast as the rest of the surgery in the mouth and neck area. Obviously it was just going to take a little longer.

The next step was radiotherapy – much sooner than I expected. An appointment was arranged for me to visit the Oncology Department and to meet Dr Macmillan again, the consultant oncologist at Northampton General Hospital. I would be having radiation treatment for five days a week for six weeks. "Great," I remember thinking. "Why now?" Just when I was feeling so much better.

Why sculptor Bunny cast Carol's features

IT ONLY became apparent to me, when Carol was recovering from surgery that the specialists' term, 'belt and braces,' meant that there were two very distinct phases of treatment to undergo. Because of our total involvement with Carol's physical recovery, the inevitable encroachment of radiotherapy had become somewhat blurred – almost forgotten.

Our first introduction to the Radiotherapy Department involved a tour of the actual unit housing the remedial machinery. It was explained, in quite simple terms, that a beam of electrons would be fired at precise points into Carol's throat and effectively zap any remaining cancerous cells. Simple. They would control the beam in three ways. Firstly, a protective mask would be made of Carol's head and neck. Holes would be cut into it in the appropriate places to allow the beam to enter. Secondly, the beam had to pass through a gridded tray, which was attached to the machine onto which were strategically placed blocks of lead.

This prevented the beam from indiscriminately spreading its dangerous waves. Thirdly, the intensity of the beam could be controlled. It all sounded like a very primitive method even though the actual machinery looked frighteningly high tech. But so much has changed and improved again in the years since then.

Carol duly had her mask made which involved taking a fine plaster cast of her head and neck. Thankfully I accompanied Carol to the studio because whatever wonderful qualities nurses have, they are not sculptors or mould-makers. I, however, was!

So rather bizarrely I began to cast Carol's features under the watchful and hopefully impressed eyes of the staff. Even so, Carol said it wasn't a pleasant experience being encased in plaster, but I think she felt confident about my involvement.

And why Carol keeps the mask in her cupboard

MAKING the mask was certainly quite an experience. Bunny's enthusiastic involvement was reassuring yet I couldn't help nervously wondering if maybe he was nostalgically recapturing his student life as a sculptor. He was obviously very pleased with the final results.

It was a horrid claustrophobic event and I was thankful when it was over. Strangely enough, I have kept the mask. It's buried in a cupboard and I thought maybe one day I could paint it in very bright colours. But I haven't as yet and I probably never will although I did hear of another patient who made her mask into a hanging basket.

When the mask was ready, there were lots of visits to have it fitted correctly on my face and neck. Making marks, dots, and crosses on the mask to verify exactly and precisely where the radiation beams would penetrate my face and neck. Each time I was lying on a special table with my head, neck and shoulders clamped down inside the mask.

I had to lie perfectly still and breathe through a straw in my mouth and with claustrophobia setting in I devised a way to cope with my ever-rising panic. I would dream about all sorts of things and that certainly helped. I was always being ticked off at school for dreaming and it's funny to think how helpful it had now become.

When radiotherapy started, it was a journey into another unfamiliar world, which slowly took its own toll.

Clare – on the grim reality of cancer

MUMMY told me she had cancer but surely only other people get cancer. Not vivacious, beautiful, caring Mummy – my best friend. I had to be strong but how can you be strong when you are unclear as to what has just hit your life?

My thoughts, I'm afraid, were not good ones. My memories of that time are of intense anger and betrayal. This 'thing' had come and taken my Mum.

Do you know how hard it is to watch the person you love most in the world become so scared and yet have to be so strong at the same time? To watch her cope somehow with simple everyday tasks, to feed your Mum through a tube into her stomach, to watch her burn during her radiotherapy treatment, to see her lose lots of her lovely curly hair and cope with difficulty when trying to swallow pureed food after six weeks of radiation?

This is the reality of cancer. But now, having recovered, once again, my best friend is back. My Mum is bossing me around and never stops chatting, laughing and most of all, doing what we do best – shopping!

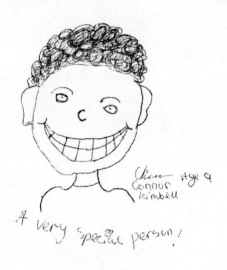

Connor Kimbell Age 9

A very special person!

Carol recalls her radiotherapy

THE radiotherapy lasted five days a week for six weeks. Bunny, or my friend Jane Garrard, who gave endless time to support me, always accompanied me. Clare also helped when she could, sometimes bringing my young grandson

Connor along. This helped cheer up other patients in the waiting room as they watched his mischievous antics.

We would wait in a small room and Jane asked if she could see the room where I was to be treated as it helped her understand what I was going through. Clare and Bunny did the same, fascinated by the whole procedure.

The room was large, with a special bench in the middle. I would climb up on it and lie flat, my body arranged by the technicians. The mask would be fitted over my head and shoulders and bolted down to the bench. My upper chest had been marked by two indelible dots to be used as a locater. I still have these marks today.

The technicians would then disappear behind some glass in an anteroom, from where they would activate the beams. The treatment is quite painless but as it continues over the weeks, other effects begin to kick in.

I was advised during treatment not to wash my face and neck area but to just dab gently with a moist sponge. I had to be careful when washing my hair and wear no make-up or perfume and I imagine that for men, shaving would be very difficult.

The days were sunny and I would sit in the garden, in the shade, watching Connor play in his paddling pool and enjoying the summer. It was a time for reflection – a quiet time. Jane continued to drive me to hospital for treatment, reassuring me and keeping my spirits up with lots of chatty gossip. I am eternally grateful to her.

By the third or fourth week I began to feel quite nauseous and extremely tired. At this point I was prescribed anti-sickness pills to take before each session of radiation and these did help. My hair was thinner than ever and so was I – not the best way for anyone to lose weight. Thank God I still had Billy the PEG, as at this stage I couldn't eat. Even drinking fluids was extremely difficult. All the good healthy meals Peggy had made during my recuperation were proving beneficial now. My mouth was sore because I was being burned and it erupted in ulcers, which were extremely painful. This was not a good time and I was plunged into the depths of self-pity.

But then miraculously, the turning point came. I had an overwhelming desire to eat an onion omelette. This was quite a challenge. It ended up a sloppy mess, but joy of joys, I was able to swallow a little down. I probably couldn't taste much of it, because by this time, as all those who have had radiotherapy treatment know, the taste buds have been hammered and everything tastes like diesel oil – horrid.

I had discovered I could now make some sloppy foods go down with plenty of milk drunk at the same time. It often resulted in lots of choking but I was getting there.

The treatment finally came to an end and I had a friend's wedding to look forward to, an important marker in my journey. I dressed up, wearing a pink dress and jacket and a large pink hat with one of Elsa's floaty chiffon scarves wrapped loosely around my neck. The burning from radiation does carry on afterwards for a while, somewhat similar to cooking with a microwave oven. My neck was rather black and sore and I put lashings of Vitamin E cream on which seemed to improve the burned area a lot. It was quite remarkable how quickly my skin healed and the wedding was such a happy day. Everyone greeted me so warmly and enthusiastically; I really felt more like my old self again.

I can't thank Dr Macmillan and the Oncology staff enough. They had always been there for me, helping and encouraging me all the way.

And now I'm feeling so much better

SEPTEMBER was soon approaching and I was recovering fast from the essential radiotherapy treatment. I still felt very tired, even exhausted at times. But I knew I would improve as I regained my strength.

My speech was not good and at times caused much confusion and hilarity. I would say something to someone and the answer would be nothing remotely like the one I anticipated. I often wondered what on earth they thought I had said, but didn't like to ask.

I had difficulty pronouncing certain syllables and consonants, making my visits to speech therapy more important than ever after being zapped for six weeks with radiation rays. I couldn't pronounce Ks and Gs due to losing one third of my tongue. Words such as *eggs* and *dogs* would become *ebbs* and *dobs*. A *drink* would become *gink* and I am still teased unmercifully about *ginks*.

In fact *ginks* has become part of the family vocabulary. Poor old *Grandpa* became *vampire* and although I know this is not a very common word, *cuckoo* became *hookoo*, a new breed of bird. John Shephard, my brother-in-law, often persuaded me to try to pronounce *cuckoo*, and much delighted by *hookoo*, we would end up in fits of giggles.

47

Unfortunately, the jaw tends to seize up. I had to try to widen it every day by performing various jaw and tongue exercises and by building up more and more wooden spatulas clenched between my teeth. I was supposed to get twenty plus in eventually, but I'm ashamed to say I don't think I ever reached my target. I know I still can't open my mouth very wide but I can make it wide enough to cope with visiting the dentist, eating, or brushing my teeth.

I watch in amazement how wide people open their mouths when they eat their food. How easy it looks and just how easy it is not for those who have had mouth cancer.

My grandson recently asked me to stick my tongue out. "I can't," I said. After much persuasion, I eventually managed the tip only. "Hurrah," he cried, "Will you do that for all my friends?" We both collapsed with much merriment.

I laughed and thought how strange it all was. So many things are so different and yet I'm still the same person. I can't whistle any more, but I can still sing, which I do find odd.

Feeling confident enough, I eventually returned to work on a part-time basis. I was glad to be back with all my workmates again. We used to have such fun and laughter and I had missed them all terribly. I was longing to paint ceramics and be creative. My right hand was fine by now but my left hand had less mobility. The area, where the flap/graft was, had taken longer to heal than expected and I had to return to NGH for further treatment by Sister Jane Bradley. I also had to wear a splint for a while to keep the fingers and thumb straight. My visits to the Physiotherapy Department were also an on-going occurrence and my neck, shoulders and arm had to be exercised regularly to increase mobility.

Back at work, I was greeted by all my colleagues and friends, Jim, Eline, Tim, Gabi, Jo and my own team, Nicky, Nic, Jenny, Alison and Diane. Sadly this didn't last too long for the company I had worked with for ten years fell into liquidation which was a very heavy blow.

In fact 1998 was my Annus Horribilis, because we had many tragedies that year. Friends asked how I coped, but it's nothing to do with coping. Things happen and we have to deal with them somehow.

Bunny's mother, who had some months earlier been diagnosed with a brain tumour, died very suddenly. This was catastrophic for Bunny and our roles reversed, with me trying to help him with his grief.

Within a month, my very dear friend Lynne, an art student contemporary from the heady 60s, was rushed into Intensive Care where she later died. She acquired a splinter in her finger, while gardening, that began to poison her blood stream, ending in a painful death. She had Tetanus, otherwise known as Lockjaw. This was indeed a terrible time and it made me really concentrate on living every moment to the full. Why had I been so incredibly lucky to survive and why did Bunny's Mum and Lynne die so tragically?

Mr Pratt advised us to have a holiday and Bunny and I decided to travel to Orkney, stopping at Edinburgh to visit my sister, Inga. Then we drove to the west coast of Scotland and stayed at The Loch Melfort Hotel with stunning views over the Isle of Jura. By this time it was well into autumn and the colours were glorious. It was now five months after my op and I still had the PEG.

Being adventurous that night at dinner, I tried to manage some soup – a potage. After explaining to the chef what was required, I was given the royal treatment. I had pureed vegetables and pureed fish, washed and gulped down slowly with copious amounts of water. I had also discovered by this time that mashed potato was a basic need as a carrier to swallow other foods. I did manage a little bit and was thrilled. This was my first night out eating with other people present and I don't think I disgraced myself. I remember finishing off with a very light lemon mousse and cream and it was heaven.

Another great coup was being able to drink wine, again. Only a little, but about one third wine and two thirds cold, still water. To this day, I cannot drink wine without filling the glass half full of water. The acidity in my mouth is too much, thanks to the results of radiation.

On we went up to Scrabster outside Thurso, sailing over the Pentland Firth to Stromness and arriving at my aunt's home near Kirkwall. Aunty Lib was absolutely over the moon to see us, spoiling and fussing over me. Her dry wit and humour ever present, making us feel at home. In fact this *was*, in a sense, home for me. This was the house where our very large extended family spent our summer holidays every year when we were young. This was the house my grandfather built and where my mother was born. Other cousins, Peter and Anne, Karen and Stan, all insisted we stay with them too. We were welcomed back into the fold.

Something else happened while we were there. We bought a peedie (Orkney word for *small*) house in Stromness. I couldn't believe our luck. This was something I had always longed for and it's right by the sea, overlooking the harbour and has the most wonderful view. Our journey north was like a beacon of light, pulling and guiding us through all those bad times we had endured. We still have the house and stay there as often as we can.

Returning home to Boughton, we had much to plan. Christmas was coming, we had plans to make for the new house in Orkney and most important of all, our wedding for the following Spring.

Tragedy follows our happy Christmas

CHRISTMAS was a time for us all to be together. Only James was missing, still out in Australia. What a joy it was to be at home and immediately after Christmas, Bunny and Roger packed a load of furniture and bedding into a large transit van we had hired to transport everything up to our new holiday house in Orkney. They left before New Year and drove 650 miles north, catching the ferry to Stromness.

Everything seemed to be going fine when tragedy struck. Roger's son Daniel was reported missing over New Year and Roger hurried south to hear the tragic news of his son's death. This was a dreadful time. Roger, who had helped us so much during our difficult times had also been a cancer patient. He had had cancer of the throat a few years before and had recovered from his surgery, coping with his speech problems amazingly well. Roger is a Graphic Artist and he has designed the book cover for us together with illustrations for some of the recipes. He has helped us enormously through good times and bad. He was to be Bunny's best man for our wedding and we can never thank him enough.

How I had to create
my own job

TIME moved on and I no longer had a job, due to being made redundant. I went to the Job Centre to sign on for the first time in my life and I was told I wasn't fit for a job because no one could understand a word I was saying.

I was shocked. Apparently in most jobs speaking on the phone would be essential. This was quite a stumbling block, but it made me angry. I had lots of fight in me and this time I was going to do something positive.

We had a barn in the garden and Bunny built a ceramic decorating studio for me, complete with a kiln. I now had the ability to continue with my creative work and found this a great confidence booster and an ideal therapy. This was, and still is, my salvation, offering a quieter environment than my former job and one I felt I was in charge of. I began to paint, glaze and fire bowls, jugs, mugs and tiles and encouraged friends to join me. We enjoyed painting days together and still do and I sell my work, not only locally but on a much wider basis around the country. I am very lucky to enjoy such creativity and it has helped me enormously to a speedy recovery.

The next major step was having Billy the PEG removed. I felt a little nervous about living without him, but this was the way forward. I was managing to cope with certain foods at home like the pureed drink Fortisips, porridge or ReadyBrek. Mashed up banana, yoghurts and mashed potato were a constant standby, including a glass of wine, albeit watered down.

My taste buds seemed to be returning but not everyone recovers at the same pace or in the same way. I can't eat a sandwich of any description and I can't eat curry although I know plenty of others who can. Whereas I can enjoy taste again, for some this is not always possible. Anything fizzy is lethal for me but it's manageable for many others. This is a learning curve and a lot is discovered by trial and error.

I hope to pass on what I have learned in the last eight years but I can only say if it's all right for me. Hopefully, however, it will be of some help with the recipes and tips in a later chapter together with advice from the hospital dietician.

My visits to Mr Pratt still continued and at one check-up it was discovered that I had a slight problem. One of the metal plates in my lower jaw had moved and was possibly fractured. Arrangements were made for more surgery to have the offending plate removed. And since the scar tissue under my chin was so tight, I was to have more surgery there too. I presumed this would be rather like a 'nip and tuck' procedure and this proved to be a great improvement. At last I could throw my head back and turn it left and right with more mobility. I no longer had the double chin caused by fluid build-up following my lymph gland removal and I felt fantastic.

The stitches came out just in time. Bunny and I were going to be married in Orkney with the ceremony in my aunt's house where my mother had been born. The date was fixed for June 2, my mother's birthday.

We stayed in our peedie house where we met all my family coming up from the south, including two very close friends John and Joy who had come up especially to be with us and of course Roger, our best man. Best of all, my son James arrived after spending nearly a year away in Australia. I was overjoyed to see him.

James returns to find Carol looking good

I WANTED to make it a surprise for Mum's wedding but the secret was out early on and the biggest shock my family received on my return was my bleached blond hair colour and phoney eyebrow piercing.

I had been away in Australia for almost a year, having left when Mum was out of hospital recovering but still before her radiotherapy. The decision to go ahead with this pre-booked expedition was difficult and only taken after strong assurances from Mum and support from my family.

It was a good job I went for destiny certainly played its part when I met Melissa, my future wife, in Australia. My life was changing rapidly but after a year's travelling with constant communication but no visual contact, my mind was awash with images and concerns over Mum's recovery and condition.

This all evaporated in an instant the moment I was reunited with her and Bunny at the cottage in Orkney. She looked fantastic and although she'd lost some weight, she was every bit the mother I remembered and loved. It was a shame her jokes hadn't improved very much, but two days later Alastair and I gave Mum away at her wedding – a fantastic end to a traumatic year.

Bunny recalls the
wedding day

ORKNEY is not exactly renowned for its good weather. The Orcadians call it 'the blink' – a beautifully succinct description. By way of explanation, if you blink three times, then you can expect rain, wind or sun, or any other combination. Orkney days just entail a lot of blinking, really.

The day before the wedding was indeed a mixture of wind and rain, but we were so busy making sure that friends and relations had arrived safely and knew the arrangements for the following day, that we hardly noticed it.

In the evening Carol stayed with Judy, John and Elsa at Little Bu, another family home, and Roger Wilkin, my best man, and I stayed in our little house, facing the harbour in Stromness. We raised our whisky glasses to the memory of important people and retired early to bed, hoping for a good start the following morning.

It was a crystal clear day with bright sunshine and no wind. I was immediately connected to the power of prayer. Roger and I got ready and drove across the island to the Bungalow, a family house owned by Aunty Lib where the wedding was to take place.

We arrived early and as we nervously talked to Lib, the minister arrived. We were all standing around the kitchen table and Lib announced she was making tea 'to help calm our nerves a little'. Whereupon Roger dug deep into the inside of his jacket and produced a quarter bottle of Highland Park whisky.

Two things seemed to happen simultaneously. The tea cups magically transformed into glasses and nervousness was replaced by laughter. The four of us drank two drams each before the guests arrived, a very happy beginning to a wonderful day.

A wonderful recipe for recovery

THE big day arrived and the weather was beautiful – blue skies and not a cloud in sight. And for once it was warm. Alastair and James gave me away and Clare and Connor were close by my side. It was a memorable and happy occasion and Bunny and I were deeply moved as we said our vows.

After the ceremony we went on to my cousins Peter and Anne's house in Kirkwall, where more guests joined us for food and dancing. Later that night Bunny and I literally sailed away to another small island called Shapinsay where we stayed in Balfour Castle. It had been a very special day.

Eventually we came down to earth, making our way home to Boughton. A week later we had a huge celebration party in a marquee in John and Judy's garden in Boughton. We invited all our friends to join us that night and it was a magical evening. This also had a special meaning, as this was the home where I had spent my childhood and teenage years. Bunny and I were so happy and it was a wonderful recipe for recovery.

Often I find myself thinking back to childhood memories for we had a very happy upbringing, clothed in security and love. We were always surrounded by lots of animals, boxer dogs, rabbits, guinea pigs, Micky the pony and even a pet pig called Wiggy. My father was a well-known Veterinary Surgeon, with a large practice for farm animals and domestic pets. My mother had worked as a Bacteriologist in her earlier years but once her family arrived, she was always there for us at home, her deep family roots giving us all a very solid upbringing.

I am sure this gift of love, which our parents passed on to the three of us, has sustained my efforts to keep going during those weeks of fright and fear of the unknown. I wish I could tell them now how much their strength has helped me although I'm thankful they didn't have to endure what we all went through. But I know they were there for me in so many other ways.

How Carol found
some support

AS TIME moved on I became increasingly aware that, apart from my regular check-ups, there was very little back-up or therapy for me. I had not met anyone else who had experienced mouth cancer.

I had read John Diamond's book, *C – Because Cowards Get Cancer Too*, but still felt isolated. I couldn't relate to anyone else about how I really felt and though my family were ever supportive, I desperately needed a bit more.

Mr Pratt agreed there was a lack of immediate contact and support for patients recovering from mouth, head and neck cancers and suggested I meet another patient, also in remission, who was recovering from mouth cancer. Her name was Valerie Johal and I met her by arrangement in the

Maxillofacial department. We could hardly believe it but we really related to each other.

This is how our support group was born with Valerie and I meeting at the hospital about once a month with Sister Jane Bradley acting as facilitator. Eventually we grew into a larger support group until it became the registered charity FACEFAX.

Anne Hicks, who is highly qualified as our Maxillofacial Clinical Nurse Specialist, acts as our facilitator now. She is extremely patient, giving up much of her precious time and always full of advice. She listens carefully to all we have to say and must sometimes leave with a raging headache. But we couldn't do without her.

Mighty oaks from little acorns grow and Valerie and I are proud of our achievement. We have many others on board now, actively working hard to achieve more awareness of this still little known cancer where early diagnosis is so essential.

I met my fellow author, Ann Bennett, at one of our meetings in 2005 and we immediately hit it off, both recognising certain needs within the support group. We were both able to laugh at ourselves and the awful predicaments we sometimes get into. This was a breath of fresh air and a firm friendship developed.

I was in remission for two years, although I'm never quite sure what that means exactly. Did I still have cancer or not? Two years seems to be a magical number and during that time I learned that Mr Pratt was leaving.

I did panic at first as my safety net was being removed and this was an anxious time. But I was soon put in the safe and capable hands of Mr Smith who had also been present at my big op. I hadn't seen him much until now but I was much re-assured by his quiet, caring manner and even now I have regular six-monthly check-ups. Five years is the next magical number and then we are let off the hook. I decided to keep up with the six monthly check-ups and still see Mr Smith.

Before concluding, I must mention another special friend who has played a big role in my journey, Elke from Prussia. She and I were both at art school together many years ago and she married Malcolm Pollard, who in those days was our very handsome young sculpture lecturer.

Dear Malcolm died a few years ago within four months of diagnosis of cancer of the oesophagus, never having smoked in his life. Elke and I keep in close contact and we often paint together. They are happy days and she is a 'darlink' (Elke's famous pronunciation of her favourite word.) She has very kindly illustrated our stories in this book and I thank her so much. I must also thank my cousin Elsa, who has typed and proof-read my manuscript.

Where I am is here

THIS heading is a line written by my mother's cousin Margaret Tait in her book, *Subjects and Sequences*. It tells of her work as a film director and poet and it seems rather appropriate at this point in the journey.

It had a hugely enjoyable stopping place in 2004 when many of my friends in Boughton village gathered together to raise money for our local Cynthia Spencer Hospice. We did the Calendar Girl thing and it was enormous fun.

I was voted as Cover Girl for our very tasteful calendar of glamorous naked ladies and this was a huge honour for me. We raised a significant amount of money in a relatively short space of time. All those who participated had been affected by cancer in some way. Marie Boullemier, our friend and neighbour was Miss November, having had cancer herself.

I have a very full life. My ceramic work continues and hopefully always will. My aunt and Godmother Dorothy, known as Dor, kindled my interest in ceramics originally. She herself was a painter with a great interest in ceramics and had her own studio in Oxfordshire. I use her kiln in my present studio now.

It did take at least two years to recover from surgery and radiotherapy treatments and I don't think that at the time I realised this. It's only now, looking back that I can see how far I've travelled. I still get tired but that's just age and I have much more energy these days.

Someone asked me the other day, "So are you over it now?" Cured, I suppose he meant. I thought for a moment and replied, "You learn to live with it – it never entirely leaves you." This must have shocked him, because he deduced that in that case, I must still have cancer.

But no – I am better now. It is eight years on but any little ache or pain in the head or neck and mouth area will transport me right back to the point of alarm, worry, and what if? I don't suppose anyone who has had cancer will fail to understand this for we all try to adjust to live alongside these fears with trust and hope for the future.

I have quite a lisp still and when I get tired it becomes more pronounced. But hey – I'm here. I still have to eat foods with lots of sauces or gravies and the inevitable mashed potato. Friends are so good about this and always make allowances by asking what I can manage and offering extra sauces.

I love all kinds of fish and eat plenty of chicken and vegetables and I have to say I adore my puddings. I have to watch this carefully as too many sweet things are not good for my teeth. I did smoke before I had cancer, but gave it up immediately I was diagnosed, leaving me with the legacy of my sweet tooth.

I have a survival kit that I carry around with me everywhere I go. A bottle of water, toothbrush, saliva spray or gel and sometimes chewing gum – sugar free of course. Without the water or gel or gum my mouth would completely dry up. I don't think I would survive long in a desert and I have listed the toothpaste, gel etc in the Therapies section.

This coming Christmas will be a very special time. I will have all my family with me, including grandchildren and more grandchildren on the way. Inga and Judy and their families will be with us too.

Last but not least, Bunny who has been a Trojan, working endlessly, day and night, on the book project. What can I say – he is my soul mate, my hero.

My experience has altered my personal perspectives in a way I cannot ignore. I try to get as much out of my life as possible but this is not always easy. I realise Ann and I have two very different stories but without exception we have one fundamental belief in common. That is to fight, believe in our strength and hope for the future. As my sister

Judy quoted in the Boughton Calendar, for 'tomorrow and tomorrow and tomorrow'.

Carol Dunstone, July 2006

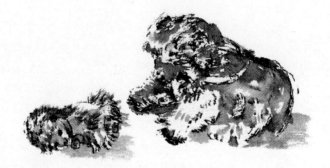

CHAPTER THREE

Ann's Story

WHEN one of life's biggest challenges arrived completely out of the blue, the initial shock of my cancer diagnosis rocked my world and that of everyone close to me.

But time doesn't stand still and in between hospital visits, preparing for a nine hour operation and not feeling particularly fit, I had a choice. Either I lived in fear and anger or I prepared to fight, not really knowing the outcome. So all in all, it was pretty scary.

What I *do* know is how important other people are at such times. I had the help of a caring medical team and the wonderful love and support of my family and friends including a text from my son that I will cherish forever.

"Do not worry Mum, it will be a false alarm. You will be alright. And if it's not, you'll still be alright and Dad and I love you very much x"

Among other supporters was my cousin Vicky Golding, who had lost her own mother to cancer at the age of nine.

She travelled down from Yorkshire to see me during the early days of her pregnancy. I hope that all of the above mentioned believe me when I say that I will never forget them and each individual act of kindness. I did my best to put the smile back on their faces and looked for ways to cope.

When you are a communicator and you're told you won't be able to speak for a while; and that when you do, nobody can tell you how you are going to sound, it's rather daunting. When you love your food and you are told you will be fed through a 'PEG' (a feeding tube inserted directly into the stomach 10 days before the operation) you know it's not going to be easy.

My friend Yvonne Miller is also a counsellor and is used to liasing with doctors and patients. So before surgery she very kindly offered to give up her working time for my appointments. She was supporting not only me, because I just couldn't take it all in, but also my husband Michael and my sister Sarah Erickson who also attended the pre-op hospital appointments. She was also invaluable in making telephone calls to family and friends, especially when I was unable to talk.

I was aware that for some people there is never a good time to be ill and the timing for my husband's family wasn't good. My sister-in-law had died of cancer in the same week ten years earlier and I couldn't help thinking about them. I asked my husband not to tell them and resolved to fight and stay positive.

It is unrealistic to think that you can be positive all the time so you need to give yourself time to reflect, have a good cry and allow yourself space to think about how you're going to 'face the fear'. And for me, how to turn it round and grasp what could lie ahead, based on the facts and possibilities I had been given by the medics. As a Holistic/Complementary therapist with over 14 years' experience, which included running my own practice involving hypnotherapy, Reiki and spiritual healing, I was fortunate in knowing where to go for support. No matter how much knowledge one has gained through life, nobody can do it all on their own.

I thought sharing my experiences in a book would be a good idea and hopefully a help to others. I asked Carol Dunstone if she would like to join me in putting it together, especially as our experiences had been so different. We originally talked about a recipe book made up of tried and tested meals for people like ourselves, but I felt there was room to expand the book from what we had learned. And quite frankly, I did not have as much knowledge as Carol in creating the varied and interesting menus that prevent one getting bored and overwhelmed by the restrictions. Carol's operation was eight years ago in 1998 and she had been battling with the challenge long before I did so I must thank her and her kind friends in the art world who are responsible for the illustrations. I hope readers enjoy them as much as I do.

The meaning of Trilogy

I WANTED to make sense of what had happened to me, turn the experience round and do something positive with it; in other words, not to waste the experience but to allow myself to move on:

The book's title, *A Trilogy of Mind, Body & Spirit*, came about because there are three strands to getting over the ordeal that Carol and I went through.

The Mind – because as a hypnotherapist, I understand the power of positive thinking, and the important part the mind plays in handling a crisis and not giving up;

The Body – which includes ideas on clothing, massage, beauty tips and recipes;

The Spirit – whether it be prayer, Reiki, spiritual healing, Buddhist philosophy, a respect for a higher power, or a combination of all belief systems, it does not matter. It will all help. I know this from personal experience, although I am cautious not to ever use the word 'cure'. At the end of the day, whatever will be will be. But at least you can say you tried.

I have been digressing so I must now return to my journey. With two weeks to go between diagnosis and the operation, I assessed my wardrobe without taking into account that I would lose a stone in weight and that clothes with waists would be difficult because of the PEG. As my family and friends know, I will always find a good excuse to shop and clothes are usually a great source of pleasure for me. But this was different.

My first tip therefore, is to change your mind-set and think 'comfortable' (something which I became well practised at). And once the PEG is inserted, buy a few drawstring trousers. Thank goodness there are some fashionable ones around! However I did forget that my arm would be in plaster due to the reconstructive surgery needed to rebuild the inside of my mouth.

To be perfectly honest, I could not get my head around this significant part of the process, probably because I did not want to. Was this my stubborn streak coming out? I do remember, though, being asked which arm I would like them to use. "Wow! I have a choice!" Joking apart, this is actually vital. You wouldn't want your writing hand immobilised because when you're unable to speak, writing is the only way you'll be able to communicate. I was also told that I would not be able to move my arm for at least two weeks and that it would take some time to heal.

Now I realise how very important and clever this part of the operation is and how proud and grateful I feel towards the surgeons. The reconstructive surgery consists of a piece of tissue with an artery and a vein attached, which is removed from another part of the body (in my case, my arm). This is called a 'free flap' and the tissue is transplanted into your mouth to fill the gap left by the removal of the cancer (in my case the floor of my mouth on the right hand side). In truth, I have only just read up on this. Until now, a convenient 'blonde moment' would occur if anybody asked me about the reconstruction and these moments come in useful when you don't want to deal with something

Michael 'operates'
on my new tops

AFTER the operation, Michael and I realised that my tops were not suitable so he went shopping and came back with some very stylish ones. Under normal circumstances, I would have been delighted and very impressed, but the sleeve on the 'flap' arm was difficult to put on and in his frustration, bless him, Michael borrowed a pair of scissors from the nurses and literally chopped the offending sleeves off all three tops leaving jagged, fraying edges. I think that was the last straw during a time that was very difficult for him. Or perhaps he thought he was still in the army and it was time to improvise.

I tried to smile in appreciation and two days later, a nurse tidied up the sleeves the best she could. We were very conscious of not wanting to offend Michael and it still makes me laugh to this day. Our friends Stephanie and David Tuckley in Devon sent a sexy red nightdress for a laugh and I just thought, "Feeling ready to wear that is a target I want to reach as soon as I can."

The next thing I turned my attention to was my face. I wasn't sure what was going to be cut; it very much depended on whether or not the cancer had gone into my jaw. We would not know until the operation. So in preparation, I concentrated on the eye area, feeling it would be fairly safe to do so. I went to my friends at Windmills, a unisex salon in Duston, Northampton for hair, beauty and holistic treatments. They took me under their wing and gave me the works. I had my eyebrows and lashes tinted to give definition because I anticipated that putting on make-up might be a challenge when one arm is in plaster.

I did put on some lipstick towards the end of my stay in hospital, although I rather wish I hadn't. My son Mark wasn't impressed as my face was swollen and my hands so shaky that I missed my lips. He helped me reapply it and at least we had a good laugh about it. I was not going to be beaten but applying lipstick felt like hard work and as I didn't want a repeat performance, I didn't bother again until much later on in my recovery.

It had been quite an eventful day and the lipstick was, in fact, representing what was in my head. I felt it was time to move on. After all, it was nine days after surgery and I did not want to start feeling sorry for myself as this is not a path I'd recommend.

I'd had the tracheostomy (a breathing-tube inserted directly into my windpipe at the front of my neck) removed. This is usually left in for anything from two to seven days and mine had been in for five. While this is in place, you are not able to talk and when the tracheostomy is removed you are so apprehensive.

Mr Colin Harrop, my consultant was full of encouragement and I thought, "If he thinks I can talk, I'll have a go". Michael said I sounded like Darth Vader and in hindsight, I must apologise to patients around me who must have thought I was making some very odd sounds. I'd discovered how to project my voice from the back of my throat like opera singers and actors are trained to do and this helped me. Coincidentally, my mother was an amateur opera singer and as a child in Swindon I spent many hours backstage at the theatre, watching her perform. So perhaps subconsciously I knew what to do.

I would just like to add that for a small child, being surrounded by strong singing voices and seeing all these grand theatrical outfits and heavy make-up is a bit scary but by using this technique, along with writing a lot of things down to fill in the gaps, I could just about make myself understood. However, this method of communicating doesn't do a lot for a humorous story and it's terribly frustrating.

Michael, meanwhile, was spending time with our friends and neighbours Sushel and Manjit Ohri. They were very supportive towards him, providing meals and visits to the swimming baths to work off the calories from Manjit's wonderful curries. With similar support from other friends, Michael was not left on his own very much.

Having been born in India, with four generations of his family serving in the British Army, Michael is drawn to anything Indian and he too makes a good curry. But when he decided to go to Birmingham to visit an Indian company that was touring the country measuring customers for made-to-measure suits, I was not very keen on this idea. Since I was not in a position to express myself very well, I decided Michael was in good hands with Sushel and Manjit, not knowing that they too shared my unease.

He duly purchased three suits and when they eventually arrived they looked like demob issue. My note-pad filled up very quickly as my Darth Vader voice was unable to portray my exact feelings.

During this time in hospital, I had a lovely male night nurse from the Caribbean. He was a fatherly figure and so sweet and patient, especially when I had to write him long messages in order to have a conversation. When I started to speak again, limited as it was, he told me that he would miss the long 'love letters'. He had such a good sense of humour which is just what you need in those long, dark hours. My poor husband thought he was going to have a nice quiet time for a while because nobody knows how long it will be before you will be able to speak or be understood. Every case is different and it's a matter of wait and see.

What a neat job, said the admiring nurses

A FEW days later, all the bits and pieces were removed from around my neck and the nurses admired Mr Harrop's handiwork. They said they'd never seen such a neat job and it was a good thing I was older because he'd followed the natural lines in my neck so the scars would not be so prominent. As I didn't have a mirror, I wasn't sure whether to laugh or cry. Had I in fact had a face-lift?

The 'lipstick day' day meant I felt more in control and even if I was wobbly I now wanted some answers. But nobody seemed able to tell me the results of my neck lymph-gland biopsy. I didn't realise it takes weeks to test these and I had thought that only one had been removed, not 'a long bundle' as one of the doctors described them. I couldn't understand the delay, but the oncologists have to be very thorough and make sure that all the cancer has been removed. This would determine whether or not I needed radiotherapy and not fully appreciating this, I accused Mr Smith, a consultant who had also been involved in my operation, of 'spin'. Poor man – you can tell I was listening to a lot of political news during this time.

I found out weeks later – not a pleasant wait for anybody – that all the cancer had been removed from my tongue. This meant that a third of my tongue had been taken away, plus the floor of my mouth on the right side, along with the lymph glands, also on the right side of my neck. This meant I wouldn't need radiotherapy and, thank God, that I did not have to have my face cut, as it had not gone into my jaw.

However, it would mean monthly check-ups for the first year, gradually spaced out over five years. Anne Hicks, the Clinical Nurse Specialist in the Maxillofacial Unit at Northampton General Hospital, assured me that the door would always be open if I had any concerns.

As I have said before, I had a wonderful NHS medical support team and this is still ongoing. I consider myself lucky to have had the cancer caught early and that I am alive. There are always people who have had more drastic measures to cope with or who live in countries where they can't afford to operate on this type of cancer. My heart goes out to them.

Although you cannot wear nail varnish prior to the operation, I would highly recommend a manicure and a pedicure. There is no reason why, when you feel up to it afterwards, you could not ask a family member or friend to put some varnish on for you. The bonus is that it will stay on longer than usual because you won't be peeling the fruit and vegetables for a while. As I keep saying, there is always a positive out of a negative and if nothing else you will benefit from the 'me time'.

Jo Wiles is a reflexologist and aromatherapist and also works from the Windmills salon. In the past, when I was running my own practice from home, she used to hire my room for her treatments and we would refer to each other and support one another with our therapies. Gentlemen, I do include you too when I talk about therapies. There are huge benefits in having some switch-off time and in my experience many people who use complementary therapies find stress levels come down and they are more able to handle day-to-day problems. All the therapists whom Carol and I mention in this book are very caring, supportive people – just what you need to see you through those challenging days.

I'd had an operation on my back three years earlier and Ilona Cydejko visits me at home once a month to keep my back muscles healthy with massage or reflexology. As a National Federation of Spiritual Healers member, I also have some spiritual healing thrown in which is an added bonus and so relaxing. Sam Murphy, a freelance hairdresser who has become a friend to the family and me over the last few years, does my hair at home, which under the circumstances, is a godsend. Nothing fazed Sam, who is not medically trained, but she was able to accommodate and overcome any problems I might have; for example bending to have my hair washed and keeping areas from getting wet, especially after the operation around my neck area. It was often quite a laugh and she shared some of my ideas for future goals and how they could be achieved. I can't thank Sam enough, not just for helping me, but also for helping me show my family and friends that I wasn't about to let myself go just because of cancer. In some ways I saw it as a challenge. And at times it still is.

Moisturising is very, very important. The nurses tell you this and not only does it help with the scars, but you can feel your skin drink the cream up. This will go on for some time. As I write this 15 months on, I religiously moisturise day and night. If I miss an application just once, the affected areas become very uncomfortable. In my case where the flap was on my arm, the throat, neck and around the tracheostomy area. I have tried lots of different creams and the most effective is Body Shop's Shea Butter for very dry skin, and Vitamin E Body Butter.

How my ordeal enriched me

AS I write this, my stomach is doing somersaults because I'm not very brave when it comes to talking about these areas. I still don't like having to look after them but if I do, they must eventually fade like the memory because even now, I can't really believe it happened to me.

However, in a very strange way, it has enriched my life through meeting new people, learning from, and experiencing new challenges and most of all, really appreciating the love and support I have received. Sometimes people say that you never know until the day you die, how rich your life really was. Hmm. I think I do. While in hospital, restless legs would drive me to despair. Lying around is not good for anybody and with a back that likes exercise, I needed some help. Because of the 'tracky' and other bits and pieces, I wasn't able to move very much for a few days. But fortunately for me, my sister and Yvonne offered to massage my legs and feet with Arnica Gel – great relief and good for a wide range of aches and pains. And of course, the bonus is that it's natural. Information on how to order Arnica is in the Contacts & Referrals chapter.

When visiting me at home, Vicki Barber, a friend who is a massage therapist and has her own practice, offered to give me a leg and foot massage as a present. It was an unexpected offer at a time when I needed help to stay positive and focused. It was a period of time that I'm sure many are familiar with after such an event. You are spending more time on your own and need to come to terms with such a life-changing situation that tends to make you feel very emotional and when you least expect it, very tearful. Thankfully it does not last.

During this time, my friends just seemed to know instinctively when and what needed doing and I was constantly amazed at their timing and their kindness, even just calling in and sorting the flowers, nothing ever seemed too much trouble.

Lots of wonderful, kind gestures were all the more appreciated as we are not a large family so friends are very important. At different stages of my progress they each came into their own. Like Julie Barnes-Ward who had nearly lost her own life four years ago and who sat holding my hand as I drifted in and out of sleep not long after the operation. I was not aware of this at the time and was only told later by my sister. Months later, Julie and her business partner, Alan Spooner, owners of *Business Times*, kindly printed a piece on FACEFAX helping to raise awareness in the business community. We in the support group all appreciated their help.

Erika Takàs, my Hungarian schoolfriend whom I'd met when I first came to Northampton at the age of 14, was, like me, an outsider who hadn't been through the Northampton school system. This brought us together all those years ago and after my operation, Erika would dash in and out between her work commitments to check I was ok and promised to build me up with her Hungarian recipes which are very tasty and could be pureed for when I came out of hospital.

She did not let me down and used ingredients from her husband Belà's allotment, which is organic. And believe me, you can tell the difference. Sadly, not long after I wrote this piece, Belà Takàs had a heart attack and died but his kindness and sincerity towards my family will never be forgotten. Since I was 16, Belà's pet name for me was Blondie, which has always made me feel young and girly. He was always encouraging me in whatever I undertook and after the funeral, Erika said to me, "You must now get on with the book because that's what Belà would have wanted."

I wasn't very big before the operation and I couldn't afford to lose the stone that I did, but once again, help came along. Frankie Button, a good friend from when we both had children at the same school 30-odd years ago, was visiting when the consultant came to see me and told me that I could have liquids.

This was on the tenth day and it became one of the most exciting days of my life as I had not been able to enjoy food for quite a while, even before the diagnosis. At the same time, Joy Ball, a retired district nurse was also visiting and that day had offered to come and look after me when I was discharged. This enabled me to leave hospital a couple of days later because somebody needed to be with me for the first few days.

Frankie and Joy discussed suitable recipes with me that could be purified. I could hardly contain myself as hunger was now a real problem due to my being dairy, soya and gluten intolerant. This was difficult for PEG feeds and the dieticians really worked at trying to get the balance right. But the thought of that nice contented 'full' feeling that I had not experienced for a long time was becoming more attractive by the minute as Frankie and Joy made plans.

Frankie creates her masterpiece

THEY both came up with all sorts of homemade soup ideas and the only down side was that I had to wait until Frankie got home to create her masterpiece. But as promised, she soon turned up with some delicious lentil soup. I was ecstatic yet very nervous about eating it. It was all finely blended and though it took me ages to drink (this is something one has to get used to and I will explain later), I felt as if I had climbed Everest.

Although I would still have to have feeds through the PEG, it was a relief to know that I would be able to consume certain foods orally and that sipping champagne, one of my visualisations, would soon become a reality.

It seemed that every time I put on the television, it was all about food, restaurants, chefs and competitions for people who wanted to be chefs. I decided that rather than becoming cross and frustrated – tempted though I was – I would write down some of their tips and suggestions for future use. It certainly paid off, even though getting to grips with a pad and pen with one hand was difficult. However, the bigger challenge was seeing the food trolley going back and forth past my hospital bed three times a day and I can

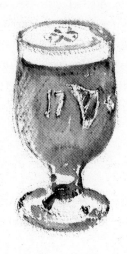

tell you that hospital food smells wonderful when you can't have any.

While you are unable to talk, it seems your hearing becomes more acute. My husband would say I have 'ears like a bat'. But regardless of Michael's kind words, when you're lying in bed unable to move very much, you can't help over-hearing other people's conversations and you tend to conjure up what the people are like and how they live their lives. You learn as much as you do by people-watching on holiday. On one occasion, two ladies were talking about having a drink, which is understandable when you're in hospital and can't have one. And how they enjoyed a pint of Guinness. They said they couldn't understand all the fuss about having a glass of champagne when, in fact, it was no more than fizzy lemonade. For some, this may well be true, but for me, not being able to respond to their comments was difficult, as I had spent a fair amount of time visualizing a glass of champagne, sitting in the sun and looking out to sea. When things were tough, this visualisation represented happy times, laughter and fun. Somehow, holding a pint of Guinness was difficult for me to imagine, but each to their own. I'm sure a pint of Guinness with its vitamin properties would do me more good but it didn't excite me despite the quarter Irish blood running through my veins. I suppose it's the sheer size of the glass that I find daunting. I'm only 4ft 11ins, but I don't think that would have put off the elves and diddy people in Ireland who are a lot smaller. As you can see, it triggered my imagination and made me giggle inside, so thank you ladies.

I am eternally grateful to all those people who intentionally and generously projected or channelled healing energy to me from all over the world. The generic term for such practice is distance or absent healing which is very effective whether the recipient is in the same room or miles away.

This was conducted in a variety of ways. Some people chose to offer good thoughts and prayers. Others used Advanced Reiki procedures to promote a positive outcome, which Christine Gould from Rei-ki Academy kindly organised and Dee Gardner from the National Federation of Spiritual Healers, head office in Sunbury-on-Thames, arranged for members to send spiritual healing. I thank you all from the bottom of my heart.

For many years when I have travelled, I have made a point of visiting a church; not only out of interest but to light candles for family and friends, especially those in trouble. Let's just say I am drawn to do it so it was lovely when I heard that the same was being done for me. I found that very touching and it made me happy. When I ran my practice, I used to tell my clients this:

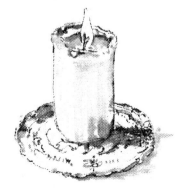

"If there is complete darkness and negativity in your world, try to imagine lighting a candle. You will find you are automatically

drawn to that light and the bigger it becomes, the lighter the feelings you had will become. See it as an energy pouring into what you had perceived to be negative. So when people feel helpless and say that there is nothing they can do, whether it be personal or global, just think of the light and the power of that light."

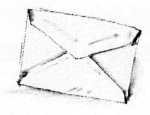

Beautiful flowers, holistic presents and cards were sent and I kept them up at home for weeks. Some made me laugh, some made me cry but they really helped me. They were healing in themselves and full of energy. I used to read them every day and felt uplifted that somebody had taken time out to remember me and send their kind thoughts. Never devalue the power of a handwritten card or letter. Technology can never replace them, however old fashioned this might sound.

Visitors who gave me a real tonic

WHILE in hospital, I had some unexpected visitors, David Samuel and his partner Guido Anino who are very funny and quite a tonic through their laughter and funny stories. They helped me forget where I was for a while and although I'm not sure that the rest of the ward appreciated their visit, for me just saying that they thought I looked great, even though I knew it wasn't true, did me the power of good and was confirmation perhaps, that the tinted eyebrows and lashes had paid off. Oh dear, what vanity. But the feel-good factor is worth striving for, even if it's in short spells.

The day my tracky was removed happened to be Bonfire Night and my son Mark and his partner Bryn walked me to the window in the George and Elizabeth ward opposite Beckets Park to watch the fireworks and see one of the Pop Idol contestants from Northampton who was singing. We certainly had a good view. After Mark and Bryn left, I felt a bit flat and my arm was becoming extremely painful. It was too early to have any painkillers so one of the nurses suggested walking down the corridor to an empty ward where there was a big television that I could watch to try to take my mind off my arm and lift my mood.

As it happened there was a programme on the history of Rock and Roll, starting in the 50s, and although this was a bit before my time in the socialising sense, I found myself dancing. I love dancing; it's great for my back and restless legs and was a brilliant distraction for my painful arm. Luckily there was nobody about, at least I hope not, but God knows what I must have looked like. Quite a sight I should think, because by then, the bruising was coming out on my face, everything hung off me and I looked as if I had been in a boxing ring rather than a dance floor. But in my head, that's precisely where I was – on the dance floor. After all, it was Saturday night and I didn't care; I was lost in a world of my own and it was great. It took my mind off my arm and I didn't need painkillers for quite some time after.

Recommended therapists' names and details are listed at the back of the book and they all showed care and compassion during the most challenging times. All are dedicated and knowledgeable in their own fields but I can hear people asking, "How can she afford to be so indulgent regarding therapies?"

Well, it's down to priorities. What's going to help and support you, bearing in mind that you won't be socialising or going out and about in the same way and eating or drinking what and when you like for a while. So the money saved can give you the tender loving care your body is crying out for and deserves. Listen to your body and you won't go far wrong, and when you're out and about on your own further down the road, people will react to you in such a lovely way which encourages you to stay focused on being positive.

However, you may also get the well-meaning person who says, "Oh, you're still well". And you can respond with a smile and say, "Yes, thank you." This did happened to me, but I had been told to expect it by Marie Boullemier, our editor's wife. She had breast cancer in 1998 but in a telephone chat just after Christmas, which I found very enlightening, her tip was: "Don't be afraid to speak to a cancer survivor."

We also talked about Christmas cards, especially to those we communicate with only once a year. I found I was unable to tie-in wishing them a happy Christmas and then updating them with my personal events, as I normally do. I was only six weeks away from the operation and felt I was unable to send them a card because my writing alone would have shown that all was not quite right in my world. So when I felt stronger and more in control, I rang them. I do hope they will forgive me for not sending a card because if I don't receive a card from someone I normally hear from, I tend to worry.

I myself count my blessings and live for the day and this is, of course, thanks to scientific research. Fortunately our chances of survival are now higher, especially if it's caught early. But the most important part is the role we ourselves play. By taking responsibility for our own health and well being, I like to think that our chances are higher.

There are no guarantees, of course. But at least you can say, "I've tried".

Ann leaves hospital and celebrates with bubbly

WHEN Michael and Sarah collected me from hospital I felt physically weak, but my mind was strong. So when a hospital manager watched me leave and said, "We don't want you coming back," I called out to him as best I could that I had no intention of returning.

I thought "What a cheek". I hadn't done all that visualisation and positive thinking to go through all that again. It's amazing how defensive one can become when one is in fighting mode and anyway, my sister had just whispered to me that a bottle of champagne was on ice, so I was definitely going home!

During one of my pre-op chats with Anne Hicks, I had asked if I would be able to have a glass of champagne so soon after leaving hospital and she said that providing my mouth felt reasonably comfortable, then why not? I discovered that one glass was pure nectar as it had been some time since my last one. I was elated at being able to drink it and in fact, it felt like an achievement. It's not that

I drink champagne daily, but when the opportunity and occasion for a celebration arises, I really enjoy it.

Having said that, I could get high on water if the atmosphere was good. Just the one glass of champagne was good though and I felt that any more would have spoilt it; anything stronger, even now, whether it be food or drink, is not very pleasant. Still, I was grateful that it did not have to be poured down the PEG; I might have experienced a nice warm glow but I prefer the more traditional way.

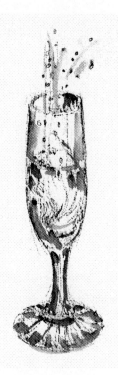

Like a baby, I was then due my next PEG feed. We were scared stiff and Michael and I had a row; this is difficult when you still can't be fully understood, but somehow we did. There were certain guidelines you had to follow and acting as nursemaid was not Michael's or Sarah's forte. To be fair, it's not mine either if put in the same position. But I was getting anxious about hygiene and the importance of using kitchen roll as I had been instructed, rather than tea cloths. Then we struggled with undoing the PEG cap. All in all it was a highly-charged first evening but I did enjoy my glass of bubbly and being able to sleep in my own bed.

The following day was just as hairy, at least until the district nurse came. She gave us what I think was some counselling and calmed the situation down. What was so nice was that all my lovely neighbours called in at an arranged time with flowers, cards and more fizz. I found that the more excited I got, the less anybody understood me so there were lots of polite nods and slightly dazed looks on faces. They will probably deny this, but I was by now used to watching expressions. I have since learned to slow down my enthusiasm to get every word out as soon as possible. My neighbour Lorraine Atherfold empathised with this and described how she sometimes finds herself cutting in because she is desperate to say something. She gets worried that if she has to wait until the other person has spoken, she will forget what she wanted to say. Lorraine reckoned this was an age thing so I stand no chance as she's younger than me. When my neighbours left I was exhausted but happy; I was alive and they all seemed to enjoy the get together.

The next day the phone was busy and Michael, in between answering the calls, had to reheat soup, specially made by our friends, and make and administer the PEG feeds. I was unable to help very much because of my arm and hand and we just thought, "Roll on Monday when our friend Joy arrives to take over." Then Michael could go back to work for a rest. That same day, my goddaughter Fern and her mother, my friend Yvonne, came to see me and they both rearranged all the flowers and checked that Michael and I were communicating!

A little bit of Joy comes into our lives

IT WAS a great relief when Monday morning arrived and we welcomed Joy with open arms. I could relax as Joy had been a district nurse and we knew I would be in good hands for the next five days. Joy and her husband Phil Ball are old friends of Michael, having met when Michael was in the army serving in Guyana. They were reunited a few years later when Michael was drinking frothy coffee in a Northampton Wimpy bar in the late 1960s and heard some familiar voices. He turned round and there sat Joy with her mother and children. Although they now lived in Wellingborough near where Phil worked, they had come to Northampton for a shopping trip and as a result they were able to pick up their friendship again. Michael made several visits to their home and when he met me, I was welcomed into the fold.

Phil and Joy now live in Huntingdon so it was a lovely surprise when Joy offered to look after me. It's quite daunting trying to work with one arm when washing and trying to keep several areas from getting wet. But we had some laughs in between the district nurse calling in. The funniest visit was when a triple order of PEG feeds arrived in several big boxes. Our home is not that small, but you couldn't move for boxes. I had thought the PEG was going to be in for six months, not six years!

On one of her visits, a district nurse said life would never be the same again and I arrogantly said, 'Oh yes it will.' I thought that with various things that life had thrown at me over the years, involving not just myself but also my family and friends, I had it taped. But you don't fully realise the impact at the time and looking back, I realise she was right. Not in an obvious way, but subtle ways of thinking have changed and I am much more aware of living and enjoying the day.

The team of district nurses from my doctor's surgery who visited me were very nice. They said that I was young to have this particular cancer but I have learned since then that mouth cancer is up by 25 per cent in young people. Raising awareness is the main reason why Carol and I wanted to write this book and have a fund raising evening. We want to raise money for a camera needed by the clinic that will help save lives by detecting the early signs of a tumour and enabling treatment to be carried out as soon as possible.

Part of enjoying the day for most of us is eating and fortunately for Michael and me, Joy thought so too. It was quite exciting wondering what creative dishes were going to be made, as they were all going to be soft blended meals for me at least. And two of her recipes are listed further on in the book.

I have not had to cook like this before, at least not since Mark was born in 1975. Now we have a bigger variety of choice and availability and because I needed building up, the dietician was monitoring my weight. Considering my gluten/dairy-free diet, she was anxious to make sure I was having enough energy-giving foods and calories. So I had vitamins and minerals in the PEG feeds and a product called Maxijul, which contained a lot of calories and could be sprinkled on everything that I could manage orally.

Fortunately, it was tasteless so it could be added to savoury or sweet dishes.

Lesley and David Gingell have become good friends over the years through our mutual friend Trudie Spicer, who moved to South Africa 12 years ago. We have a great deal in common as David also served in Guyana and Lesley, like Michael, had lived in Guildford. To top it all, David and I may well be third cousins. Is the world getting smaller, I ask myself? Or is it just proof of my belief that the people we are meant to be surrounded by will turn up in our life and enrich each other's journey? Who knows, but they do say that there is no such thing as a coincidence. Their son, Alex who had gained a Masters degree in physical chemistry, and had a personal interest in his own body shape and mass, came up with some interesting ideas for my diet. One was Coconut Connections, which supply highly nutritious ways of using coconut; one being oil that can be used to cook with. Details under Contacts & Referrals.

While Joy was with me, afternoon rests were insisted upon and quite rightly so. Lying down to sleep and rest allows the body to repair itself. This advice is not an excuse for couch potatoes though. My reward for accepting this advice was a trip with Joy to buy a new dressing gown and slippers, as mine looked a bit sorry for themselves. They had been through the mill and reminded me of the hospital. Fortunately, we had a Next nearby so we didn't have to face the crowds in town. The short outing was a real tonic and my choice fairly dramatic. That day, my friend from Seven Oaks, Yvonne Hare, or 'Little Yvonne' as we like to call her, had sent me a rather nice black scarf to encourage me to dress up, as I was very aware of my neck and wanted to keep it covered.

Scarves can play a key role for warmth and colour as well as for hiding the drama of surgery for both sexes, so stock up. Even now, I still love them and have bought lots of suitable neck dress jewellery too. My most interesting experience regarding neck attire was eight months after surgery when Yvonne's eldest son, Julian Hare, was marrying a French girl called Aurelie. We were invited to the wedding in the Loire region of France and I had planned to wear one of my many scarves. But to my horror, in my excitement I forgot to pack my scarves and neck jewellery. Michael was so good and he took me into the local town of Cholet a few hours before the wedding and we sought out a French haberdashery opposite the church where the wedding was to be held. The proprietor kindly made me a choker to match my outfit there and then. This was quite an achievement as she did not speak a word of English and I was relying on a bit of French picked up here and there. *Merci beaucoup, Madame.*

We had a fantastic time starting on the Friday evening right through to the Sunday evening. There was lots of fun and dancing and I can tell you there is nothing like a French wedding. As usual I did not want to miss anything and, as a result, I lost my voice so could not even project it. I spent half of Sunday in bed, but it was worth it. A big thank you to the family for being so kind for it had been one of my goals to make the event.

If you were lacking in self-esteem before cancer, it will certainly be a challenge to come to terms with face and body image. I used to worry about the shape of my chin. Daft I know, but since the op, the shape has changed slightly and no longer bothers me. I just think I've had a bad face-lift and laugh; it's no longer important. How many times have you heard people say, especially on the radio and television, "It's what's inside that counts" and you think, "Oh no, not that one again." But actually, it is true - if you are not happy with yourself, then no amount of external help will alter that, at least not long term. As a hypnotherapist, I would advise my clients to use the power of the mind and visualise themselves as they would like to be. Not, as in my case, as a person who has had surgery for cancer and all that that entails, but as a person who is a survivor and keen to be fit and well. The power of the mind is paramount at this time, especially for anyone who has to face a challenge in their lives. This can help you with pain by concentrating on something good and uplifting as I did in hospital.

You can use Hypno Healing techniques which I found to be invaluable; not just on myself, but also through teaching my clients how to use it. Once again this incorporated visualisation. Hypno Healing techniques were very successful with clients who were waiting to have operations – they felt that they had more power and control and that they would be able to play a part in their own healing.

I asked the anaesthetist not to discuss anything negative while I was having my operation because although I was 'asleep', my sub-conscious mind was not, and would be open to anything that was said in the operating theatre. Similarly, I did not want to discuss and go through all the nitty gritty of the operation because the whole situation was bad enough with what I did know so what purpose would it serve to know any more just a few hours before the op? I wanted to focus on being positive. I had been in this position before and had not been brave enough to tell the anaesthetist prior to my back operation that I did not want to discuss all the ins and outs when I had already been made aware of the risks by the surgeon on previous appointments. Any more 'rubberstamping' would only increase my anxiety. I realise that the medics are duty bound to discuss every procedure and some people would not have it any other way. But you do have a choice. In my case, the anaesthetist respected my wishes and we shook hands on the deal. The rest is now history.

Christine Gould, a colleague and friend has kindly submitted articles on three of the disciplines I believed in and used myself in practice. As a supporter of complementary therapies, I also respect the medical profession and have worked alongside them. The first port of call should be your doctor and if a client came to see me and had not had medical advice, I would always encourage them to seek it.

I must at this stage mention Addy Hackett, who trained with me at the Atkinson-Ball College of Hypnotherapy and who is also a consultant clinical psychologist. We shared a lot together including regression therapy and we often meet up to have deep philosophical discussions. Addy was also very supportive during the time in which I needed a lot of healing, and I know that along with others, she sent me absent healing. Words cannot express how grateful I am.

The saying 'seek and you will find' is a very good one; if I have a problem I don't give up. Michael says I am like a dog with a bone until I find the right person to help me and if you look hard enough, they will always be there. It's just a matter of having that belief and trust. Creating goals and visualizing special places in your mind's eye can also be very healing and reduce stress levels. So too, can making plans for when you feel better; in other words having a target to work towards. One of mine was driving my car which I love and enables me to be a free spirit again.

Don't waste your energy in being fearful

CHANNEL your fears into doing something positive. Don't waste that energy by being fearful. I used to say to my clients that they had done a really good job at being negative; in fact so good that they deserved a medal. So why not zap those negative thoughts with positive ones? Reframe in other words and with practice and help from your therapist, you could do equally well, if not better in your world by creating more positive thoughts.

Years ago I went on a pain management programme for my back at the Nuffield Hospital in Oxford. This involved a very intense course of physiotherapy and one of the best pieces of advice I was given was to concentrate on what I could do rather than what I could not. I also discovered that where there is a will, there is a way. It might not be the one you would have chosen or wanted, but it's amazing how effective the altering of a 'mind-set' can be. Way back in the past, I have been to all those dark places and gained absolutely nothing. You cannot change the people or circumstances which surround you but you can change your response and that in turn will help you to cope so much better. Having had two major operations within two years of each other, with lots of unexpected situations thrown in for good measure, I certainly had to walk the walk. I promise you it works. It's not easy, but the alternative is no fun. And I like fun.

Sadly, by Friday I had to let Joy go and rejoin Phil. Thank you Phil for your understanding and Joy, we enjoyed your stay with us very much and not just because you did those PEG feeds and cooked all those tasty meals.

Fortunately, I had made a decision years ago regarding the house and its physical demands and employed some help. As Michael is occupied most of the time running a company, whether it be physically or mentally, he just wants to relax with any free time, which I completely understand. The decision to employ help has been a godsend over these last few years and has enabled me to do more in my professional life than I would otherwise, so thank you Kay.

Michael and I were back to challenging times. My sister popped in while Michael was at work to do the PEG feeds, which was a laugh in itself as Sarah and I take after our father and can't stand anything medically inserted. I'm such a baby. I couldn't even look at the PEG and had to remind myself that it was a lifesaver and that some people have to rely on it permanently. I have great sympathy and respect for them. Sarah and I really struggled, whereas Michael was acting as if he was back in the army and dealt with it all very matter of fact. We got through an awful lot of kitchen towels between the three of us – thank goodness for recycling. The thought of the amount of trees we were responsible for chopping down would have induced a huge guilt-trip and I already had enough on my plate.

Towards the end of my stay in hospital, I decided that a 'bit of a do' was called for and that it would be a good goal for the following March. This gave me a few months to plan and gain strength and although I expect everyone thought I was mad, it was important to have something positive to look forward to. It was going to be a few weeks before I knew whether or not I was going to have radiotherapy and if so, I knew that the date of the event might have to be rearranged, but I was glad of the distraction. So, when therapists Jo and Vicki came to visit, I managed to put my ideas to them and said that I wanted to have a fund raising evening. My suggestion was just a small, intimate 'do' at home which would include asking my therapist friends if they would come along and give my guests ten to fifteen minute treatments in return for a donation to FACEFAX, the support group. At the time I didn't know if I wanted to be part of the group but I felt that I wanted to give something back and Anne Hicks who is chairman of this group had been so supportive.

All the therapists kindly agreed. They were fantastic and worked really hard. Sushel and Manjit played a major role, not only by making a generous donation, but by providing all the Indian snacks and helping Michael with the drinks. Fern Miller, my goddaughter, along with her mother Yvonne did very well with the raffle and the evening raised £750. Thank you to everyone who supported and took part. I really enjoyed the evening and because I did not have radiotherapy, I had plenty of time to plan. Just before the event, I had my PEG removed, thank goodness, so I was able to wear exactly what I wanted to.

This event was followed up by Janice Woods, a friend I've known since my teens. We have worked alongside each other in the newspaper industry locally and she is one of the most conscientious people I've ever known. Janice is now part of the marketing team with Northamptonshire Newspapers Ltd, publishers of the *Chronicle & Echo* and through one of our chats, it was suggested that Ruth Supple, editor of *Image* magazine might like to interview Anne Hicks and myself.

The idea was that it would help raise awareness of head, mouth and neck cancer, inform people of the support group and highlight the importance of not ignoring any symptoms that don't feel right. We were so pleased when Ruth felt that it was a worthwhile cause and I know from the feedback I have received both via the clinic and from other sources that the publication of the article has indeed helped raise awareness.

I fly out to visit Trudie – and those elephants

ALTHOUGH I had been told that I could not fly for six months, Mr Harrop agreed to me doing so at five months, just after the fundraising event. I was really keen to accept Trudie's wonderful invitation to go to South Africa as she had been unable to fly over here to see me and, in her own words, wanted to "offer her friend some TLC." This was truly worth waiting for and, bless her, she had even arranged for me to meet her doctor for her own piece of mind, even though I had said I was fine and had had a check up before I flew out. Everything was set up and Michael was going to have some peace and quiet, while accepting lots of our friends' hospitality, including Linda and Fred Cannon's, where Michael is very spoilt. So Michael would have a nice time too and he had been out to South Africa the previous year and knew that Trudie had plans for a few girly activities as well as a visit to a Safari park that had just opened and therefore wasn't commercialised.

We had some very interesting experiences and it's not surprising that the safari reserves always make you sign a disclaimer. Trudie particularly loves elephants, and took me to several different areas where they could be found. We saw an awful lot of them and one's adrenalin pumps as they are good at making their feelings clear when they decide that they have had enough of you. This is perfectly understandable, but on one occasion, I was tired and *I* had had enough of *them*. I expressed this by saying, "If I see another b***** elephant, I will scream!"

Charlotte Spicer is Trudie's daughter and my goddaughter and as I had missed her 21st birthday, it was decided, at Charlotte's request that we would go on a shopping trip and have some treats. We had a really nice time. I don't see a lot of Charlotte unless I'm in South Africa but I have a fond memory of her visiting the UK on her own when she was 12. I'd taken her to London for a long weekend to do a Reiki course and felt that the experience would enable her not only to help herself, but also her family and friends in her adopted country. Not many people in South Africa had heard of Reiki and people were very interested now that it has become much more available. As it happened, a few years later Charlotte had an experience where she was able to use her gift and help a lady who was in great pain and I'm very proud of her.

One of our visits was to the waterfront in Cape Town where a big screen was showing the Grand Prix. I knew Michael would be watching it back at home so I stopped to watch. Trudie left me for a while and I engaged in conversation with a young man to find out who was leading. It turned out that he had just moved to the Cape from England and in my eagerness to chat, I momentarily forgot about my mouth until I realized that he was struggling to understand me. The more I tried, the worse it got. He was probably the first person I had spoken to who did not know what had happened or me. I had stepped out of my comfort zone and it was a challenging moment but I knew I must not let the experience knock my confidence. But I do admit now that it made me tearful when I rejoined Trudie. I had to stay focused and really concentrate on forming my words, not speak so quickly and pretend that it was their problem, not mine. Whatever happened, for my own quality of life, it must not stop me communicating with strangers because people fascinate me and their lives are invariably interesting – particularly at Wedge View Country House and Spa where Trudie, her family and staff will treat you like royalty. I guarantee that you meet some interesting people from all over the world and this in turn helped me with some negative thoughts at this stage of communicating.

Just before I flew home Trudie, Dorothy Reyneke and I raised a glass of champagne to health and happiness as we looked across the water to Table Mountain. It was a lovely way to leave a beautiful country. It was just as well I was in fighting mode because when I got on the plane I was given an upgrade. This actually turned out to be very stressful because the reclining seat, which went into what should have been a comfortable bed, was a pain to adjust. What with being 'petite', as I prefer to say, my arm, sore tummy, neck, mouth and speech problems, I felt a nervous wreck by the time we landed. Luckily a kind gentleman helped me with my suitcase. Looking back, I must have been the entertainment because nobody seemed to mind except me. I had all sorts of men from different countries helping me – not a woman in sight. I would not normally have minded as they were quite dishy but I was feeling completely the opposite. If anybody from South African Airways reads this, please don't let it deter you from offering me an upgrade in future; I had plenty of practice the first time and I'm not likely to forget the experience!

Learning to cope with eating and talking

BACK home, I was feeling more confident, having been forced to face various fears like speaking to strangers and being on my own. Eating in front of people was a real challenge and even now, 18 months on, it still is. On the right hand side of my mouth, the removal of the tumour meant that a third of my tongue, incorporating the main nerve, was removed, plus the floor of my mouth had been rebuilt which, along with the neck surgery, creates numbness and lack of sensation in that side of my mouth and face. So when I eat, I am only aware of what is happening on the left side of my face and I feel like a hamster. A main course can take an hour to eat so you become very choosy about whom you dine with. I suggest that rather than turn invitations down and mope, particularly if you are going out with a friend and want to talk, you choose soup and sorbet or ice cream. It's not so bad if you are with a group because I have found that by saying my bit first, then concentrating on eating and listening, others will be delighted to be given a chance to talk without being interrupted by yours truly – a failure of mine. Yvonne's husband Shane Miller even suggested that I go to the restaurant earlier than everyone else, order my food and have a head start. What would you do without friends? They certainly make me laugh.

Anyway, by my eating slowly, everyone else will eventually and my friends will be aiding their digestion and possibly losing weight. Or get bored with waiting and order more food and drink, in which case, the restaurant gains. You see, there's always a positive.

Late last year, Michael took me on an 'interesting holiday' as a present for getting better. It was certainly different. We ended up spending three days in New York, and a lunchtime in Times Square. We had a meal that in England would normally be given to two people but having just spent 10 days in America I knew this was normal. As I was ploughing through my meal, one of the waiters from the other side of the room yelled out, "Hey, lady you're making real hard work of that!" I looked at Michael and thought, "This is New York." I had already had someone outside the North American Museum trying to attract my attention to buy some water by yelling, "Hey, Shorty, want some water?" I retorted under my breath that I'd have to be dying of thirst before I bought any from him – hard actually, because I did want some, but not from him.

Choking can be a problem because your ability to swallow is not as good and Michael gets very cross with me and asks why don't I cut it up smaller or have baby food. I could smack him and explain that when you have eaten one way for a great number of years, it's sometimes difficult to remember that things have changed and I'm still adjusting to that fact. I know he says it because he worries and on a normal day, when I look heavenwards at the length of time it is taking, he'll say, "Still going darling," and we both laugh. When you are out and about, people either think you've just been to the dentist or that you're sucking a sweet. But answering the phone is another challenge. If you bend your head when speaking, you suddenly find a pool of water from your mouth in front of you. So just remember to hold your head up. The saliva glands in your mouth seem to have a will of their own as some of them will have been cut.

Hunger was also quite a problem, especially in the early days due to my diet restrictions. It was highlighted when my sister and her good friend Netta Atkins and I went to see a film. I count Netta as a friend of mine too because just before I met Michael, we all shared a flat together and often reminisce about those heady days which had their highs and lows. But like all experiences in life they serve a purpose and make you what you are today. Going back to the film, it was one of my first trips out and we saw 'Ladies in Lavender'. If you've seen it, you will remember it was set in 1936, in Cornwall and all the housekeeper seemed to do was bake what we would today call good old fashioned recipes. It showed scenes of people eating big plates of this wonderful food, not worrying about calories or weight, even if the breakfast was cooked and included one of my favourites, Cornish Kippers. What really got to me was the huge 'doorsteps' of toast dripping with golden butter and homemade marmalade. What made this worse – and I blame the camera man and the producer who were obviously highly engrossed in these scenes, and for all I know did actually eat these goodies without having to share them with the audience – was that they were almost falling out of the screen. If you did not know better, you would think you too were sitting at the table. This seemed to be the case with every meal they ate, and there were quite a few. Well done to the film crew, but I do think you were a bit selfish!

I remember a few years ago, I took an Indian Head Massage course in London and was eager to practise. While working from my room at home, which isn't far from the kitchen, I heard Michael come in and, as agreed, put an Indian take-away into the oven to keep warm until I had finished. It had not occurred to me that by doing this, the smell would waft into my room and afterwards, my candidate said that she thought that I was setting the scene and imagined she was in India. I was embarrassed but we did have a laugh and I told her that it was pure coincidence. I must admit now that looking back it did not occur to me to offer her any so perhaps the previous story is karma and the universe got its own back.

Delving deeply into the mysteries of nutrition

IN those early days of convalescing, I threw myself into studying nutrition and promised my son and his partner that they would be invited regularly for Sunday lunch along with my sister-in-law, Ella Bennett.

Because of lifestyle commitments for all of us, we don't have as many of these as we would like, but when we do have one, we all appreciate it and I go completely over the top. I really enjoy cooking and it always includes a steamed syrup pudding or apple crumble with custard. We have never, or very rarely, eaten junk food or had a bad diet – at least not in my married years. When I was single and living alone I admit I did enjoy Vesta curries but then we thought that was ok and very convenient. We certainly knew how to live in those days. As I had time on my hands, I wanted to know more about nutrition relating to cancer, because as I did not smoke or drink spirits and was aware of colorants and preservatives, there were no lifestyle changes to make other than to try to improve on what I was already doing.

Having joined World Cancer Research, I know that they have a good deal of information regarding diet and health guidelines for Cancer Prevention:

1. Choose a diet rich in a variety of plant-based foods
2. Eat plenty of vegetables and fruits
3. Maintain a healthy weight and be physically active
4. Drink alcohol only in moderation, if at all
5. Select foods low in salt
6. Prepare and store food safely
7. *Do not smoke or use tobacco in any form*

(WCRF UK: www.wcrf-uk.org)

I also had a York Test to test for allergies and intolerances; the application forms can be found in some pharmacies.

Some doctors do support this test and it could be quite useful. Although I knew about my allergies and intolerances from previous blood tests at the hospital, I wanted to tidy up and when you have not eaten for a period of time, your body is finely tuned and will respond very quickly to what it does not like. (www.yorktest.com)

Recently, I read an article in a book called *'Eat and Heal'* by Dr Andrei Dracea in collaboration with Jackie Seguin, published by Bodywell. This advised against using too much sesame oil for cooking since it contains polyunsaturated fatty acids, which are suspected of causing cancer. This was very useful for me to read as unfortunately, I had until then, regularly cooked stir-fries with sesame oil, thinking I was doing the right thing.

So was this the reason for my cancer? Who knows? And I'm not going to dwell on that, but the book is very interesting and I have made a few changes since reading it. With all the information that is thrown at you, especially through the media, you could frighten yourself to death but try to take on board what feels right for you. Your body will always tell you so just listen to it as I have said before.

I remember listening to a doctor on television talking about the benefits of flaxseed oil for the prevention of cancer – that is a tip I decided to take along with manuka honey; anything is worth a try. The Daily Bread Co-operative in Northampton is very good for a variety of organic and non-organic foods which can be bought in bulk if you are not local, or don't have a lot of time. The staff has been very helpful over the years.

We had another very special wedding to go to – Nicola and Mark Steers. Nicola is very pretty and made a lovely bride. I have known Nicola and her parents, Kathy and Stuart Hills, for a number of years and they are a lovely and very thoughtful family. This was especially the case at the wedding reception. Michael and I had not, at this stage, met anyone else who had had mouth cancer but much to my surprise, the attractive lady sitting next to me had had mouth cancer seven years ago. Alexandria Ochs was Stuart's cousin and he had arranged for us to sit together. As it happened, as well as a shared medical condition, we had a lot in common. The chat we had was very uplifting and helpful, not only for me but for Michael too as this lady was so positive. We shared a few tips, one of which involved eating and trying to socialise at the same time. We both agreed that you couldn't do both, even at a wedding. But do not let it stop you from accepting invitations. That in my book would be awful.

Carol, my co-author and I, recently attended a party where we did not know anybody and ended up having the giggles because every time we went to eat, someone wanted to chat. How would they know that for us, this was quite daunting and challenging? But hopefully we did not offend anybody. If I am hungry I usually see if I can find a quiet spot and hope that nobody joins me for a little while because you really have to concentrate. Thankfully, our family and friends know this so I do not have to keep apologising. Although this is easier said than done and I get told off.

During the wedding service, Michael and I helped a mother with her two lively children and the younger of the two girls turned to me and said, "Your top is too big!" Out of the mouths of babes . . . but she *was* right. I was still thinking that I was the same size as before and this was an outfit I liked. I had gone down a size and this little girl gave me the best excuse to go out the following week and rectify this problem. So listen to your children. They can give you some good advice.

Because I had not been out very much on my own, I decided that Ossie in Northampton would be the perfect shop. This is a family run business and Gary Osborne, his daughter Sally, his sister Pat and friend Jamie were brilliant in the early days just before diagnosis when I used to pop in complaining of a painful mouth. I've always liked their clothes because they are different and they have sizes 8-16 which is perfect for me, especially having gone down a size. At the time, I was very conscious of showing my arm and neck as we were going into summer but they were all very supportive and helpful. It was particularly nice to pop in after my check-ups, even if it was just to look around. Although I admit that more often than not I would buy something. After the first 12 months, my visits to the hospital became more spaced out – once every other month. The most relieved person is Michael, knowing that my visits to Ossie will be fewer.

I find an open door
to reassurance

IT IS wonderful that the Maxillofacial clinic has said its door is always open should I need reassurance and I have, a couple of times. You can't help getting a little bit anxious prior to an appointment because however positive you are, you don't know what will be said. So thank goodness, I usually come out bouncing and retail therapy is just what is recommended, along with playing music very loudly and dancing, given the opportunity.

Roger Brown, a very old friend of Michael's lost his wife Bobbi a few months ago. Along with his other friends, we gave him support and as is often the case when someone dies, friends remember and discuss both funny and happy stories. One I did like was when Roger was sorting out Bobbi's clothes, he found at the back of the wardrobe clothes and shoes that he had never seen before. He realized that Bobbi, like a lot of ladies shop and discreetly put their purchases at the back of the wardrobe to be brought out at the appropriate time in the future stating that, "no, they are are not new, I've had them a while." I decided in her memory to call such events a 'Bobbi moment'. Roger has played a key role in helping Carol and me to raise funds for FACEFAX, which I think is marvellous bearing in mind the loss that he and his children, Ben and Olivia have had. Thank you Roger.

When I returned from South Africa, I felt that the time was right to investigate the support group. I asked Anne Hicks more about it and was assured that the group was not going to talk endlessly about their experiences which I knew was not for me. I wanted to move on and perhaps help other people to use coping strategies and stay focused in a positive way if at all possible.

It was at this stage that I met Carol Dunstone. She had had mouth cancer back in 1998 and although at the time I felt I did not want to see anyone else who had had the same experience in case it influenced me in my fight to recover, I could not bear the thought of seeing other people suffering.

I did not realise at the time that Carol was also determined to fight and stay in good health and would be a great help. When I eventually summoned up the courage to attend the support group eight months on, I was pleasantly surprised and inspired by her and we have since become good friends. It's nice to speak to someone who has experienced most of what you are going through but can have a good laugh about it too.

Last August we had a lovely evening with our friends and neighbours, Gary Cowsill and Lorraine. Gary was waiting to have an operation for bowel cancer the following week and was on a course of radiotherapy. He insisted he was fit enough to honour the dinner date but we assured him that we would come back home at any point in the evening if he did not feel well. Ironically Gary and I had arranged before I was diagnosed for the four of us to go to the theatre and see Bill Wyman and his group in concert. Unfortunately, I was taken into hospital, but rather than waste the tickets – and at the time I could not have cared less where anybody was going – Michael took Yvonne. We knew that she would enjoy it and they all had a pre-concert meal, which Michael insisted was on him. So this dinner date was arranged for when I was up to it, in between their holiday and ours.

We had a super evening and Gary was on top form; we had two bottles of fizz and the food was good. We could not believe how well Gary did, because at the beginning of the evening, none of us, including Gary, were sure as to how he would cope. Sadly, after the operation Gary had complications and died. It effected us all quite badly where we live because he was such a lovely guy, but Lorraine, Michael and I have fond memories of a great evening. Well done Gary, you were a star. At our 2006 New Year's Eve party, it was decided that we would light fireworks and have a champagne toast to Gary.

A few weeks ago, our friends Vicki and Trevor Barber came to dinner prior to an operation he needed for his heart. As usual, Trevor was upbeat and full of humour. He wanted to know more about the fund raising evening we are planning in late October and as they left, he turned around, gave me a goodbye kiss and promised a bottle of champagne as a prize. He said that as well as Vicki, who is one of the therapists working on that evening, he would also be there. We had news from Vicki a few days after the operation that Trevor did not recover. Again we could not believe it. I wanted to buy a bottle of champagne for the evening in memory of Trevor but Vicki said she had it on ice, ready and waiting. You will certainly be with us in October, Trevor along with your generous-spirited wife.

You may wonder why I have included the loss of our friends, but they and their partners played a part in my journey, and I could not pretend or deny this fact. Although painful to write about them, it was almost as if they were helping me – especially the positive way in which they were a part of this last 19 months before they went on their own special journeys. Thank you all for your support and help and may you all rest in peace.

At the time of writing I have just put a stamp on a birthday card for my cousin Vicky's son, Andrew Golding, who will be one year old. At the beginning of my journey, I mentioned that just a few days after my operation, Vicky and her lovely husband, Oscar had travelled down from Yorkshire in the early stages of her pregnancy which was a highly kept secret. But I think that they told me to give me a mega goal to concentrate on and they asked me to be there with them at the delivery. Although a daunting prospect, this was a great honour and I was also asked at a later stage if I could be there for the week following Andrew's birth when Vicky and Andrew came home. I wasn't missing all that so I'd got to get on with getting fit and well.

Vicky and I are very close because she and her brother Max Jowett lost their mother at ages nine and 11. I know their parents would be very proud of their achievements as they have done so well in their chosen professions. Despite their loss they have given Michael, Mark and me some very happy times, as well as supporting us all in more challenging ones. So last year was very special for all of us. I shall never forget the experience and happiness that new life brings, so happy first birthday, Andrew.

This journey has been a roller coaster of events one way and another, with highs and lows. It has not been possible to write about them all, but if this book just helps one person to value life, with all the twists and turns that it offers, then Carol and I will have achieved what we set out to do – to raise awareness and help save lives.

Ann Bennett, July 2006

CHAPTER FOUR
Carol's Therapists

IN this chapter I have listed the Specialist Macmillan Nurse, my nutritionist, physiotherapist, speech therapist and dentist. They have written a great deal of necessary and useful information on care for head, neck and mouth cancer patients from the point of diagnosis, through treatment and after care.

To be able to consult the Macmillan Specialist Nurse Service is a major step forwards for patients. This service didn't exist in 1998.

Advice on swallowing and eating the right foods plays a major part in nutrition and the Dietician's advice is vital.

Speech therapy and physiotherapy, from which I greatly benefited, played a major role in my case. And regular visits to the dentist are an absolute must for everyone.

An early detection of the presence of mouth cancer can indeed save lives and all the specialists listed here have enabled me to be where I am today.

Macmillan Specialist Nursing Service

By Pauline Feast

AS a Macmillan specialist nurse I am an experienced and important member of the head and neck team. I will be your key worker from the point of diagnosis continuing through your cancer journey.

As your key worker I will help to provide the best possible care information and support for patients with suspected or confirmed diagnosis of head and neck cancer.

If I am unable to support you upon diagnosis, especially those patients from Kettering and Milton Keynes, I will meet you at the first opportunity at Northampton General Hospital. I may see you with the consultant when you attend the clinic or I may visit you on the ward if you are admitted to the hospital.

So how can I help you? I can provide information about investigations, diagnosis and treatment; I can talk with you about the different treatment options including chemotherapy and radiotherapy. I can liase with your key worker and with other members of the hospital or community team about your care and support to provide a seamless service.

You can contact me at the ENT outpatients department at Northampton General Hospital NHS Trust, Cliftonville, Northampton, NN1 5BD. Tel. (01604) 523860.

My service is available Monday to Friday from 8.30am to 4.30pm. And you, members of your family, carers and friends can call for an appointment or to discuss your needs with me on the telephone with your given consent. If you have any urgent queries or problems out of office hours, contact either your GP, the district nurse or George & Elizabeth Ward, Tel (01604) 545509 / 545309.

Nutrition

By Kay Davies BSc (Hons), State Registered Dietician, Northampton General Hospital.

THERE is a general consensus that a dietician's job is to hand out milkshakes and diet sheets. However, there is much more to dieticians than you think!

Nutrition plays a vital role in aiding recovery from surgery, chemotherapy and radiotherapy for patients with head and neck cancer. Many people feel pleased to have lost a bit of weight, but this is not the time to do it. The effects of poor nutrition are extensive, influencing speed of recovery, response to treatment, wound healing, the ability of the body to fight infection and mood.

Nutritional input varies for each person but may include advice on nutritious high calorie and protein foods, obtaining an adequate intake when eating soft or liquidized meals, tube feeds (in hospital and at home) and more specific problems such as dealing with a poor appetite, a sore mouth or taste changes. Often, this involves a move away from the healthy eating principles we normally advise, to trying snacks between meals, choosing full fat and sugar versions of food and having nutritious drinks. Advice is tailored to the individual and ongoing support for people with cancer and their families and carers is essential.

With the growth of alternative therapies over recent years, complementary and alternative therapy diets are becoming something many cancer sufferers are investigating. Some of these are safe and work well alongside standard treatments. For example, having foods containing ginger to help control nausea.

However, many alternative diets lack scientific evidence to support their claims and can be expensive to follow. They may not be safe and may possibly be harmful as they are often low in calories and protein. This may therefore exacerbate weight loss in people who are already struggling.

If you are thinking of following any alternative diets or taking any nutritional supplements, please discuss them with your doctor or dietician first.

Physiotherapy

By Tracey Harris, Physiotherapy Department
Northampton General Hospital

AS a physiotherapist working in a musculoskeletal department it is unusual to get referrals for patients following major surgery to head, neck and throat region.

But when I do get one, the main aim is to assist patients in regaining as much neck and shoulder movement as possible so that they can continue with their normal lives. An assessment of the neck, shoulder and arm enables the physiotherapist to see what the main problems are post surgery.

Treatments are specific to each individual patient and patients are encouraged to do exercises at home to improve and maintain their function.

Speech and Language Therapy

By Leonie Bird and Elaine Coker

IN an ideal world the Speech and Language Therapist will be part of the Multi-disciplinary Team that you, the patient, will meet soon after your diagnosis. It may be that you will never need our input. However it can be reassuring to know that we are available to call upon if you should have problems in future, even if it is just for some simple advice or strategies to help with speech or swallowing.

After extensive surgery, particularly if a course of radiotherapy has been undertaken, Speech and Language Therapy can play an important role in recovery. Each person will be assessed and offered an individual program tailored to their particular needs. It will provide specific oral exercises, communication strategies, and, if necessary, communication aids, as well as carer support. We will work closely with the rest of the team to ensure that there is an integrated approach to your treatment.

Many people ask, "When will I talk properly again?" or, "When will I eat properly again?" Unfortunately there is no definitive answer. So many factors play a part: the extent of your particular surgery, the amount of radiotherapy you had, your healing rate, even your motivation and perseverance.

Every person is different and each will be offered help and guidance appropriate for their particular needs. In our district we have an open referral system for people with speech problems. This means that even if you have not met us before you can ring the local adult Speech and Language Therapy department and ask for help.

If you have a swallowing problem we require the referral to be made by someone in your Multi-disciplinary Team, but if you speak to us we can give you advice on how to arrange that.

Dentistry

By Waterhouse Dental Practice, Northampton

HEAD and neck surgery and radiotherapy can lead to several side effects to the mouth and soft tissues and it is advisable to seek your dentist's help on how best to look after your mouth during this time.

When you, the patient, are first diagnosed as needing surgery and radiotherapy promptly, you may find that the condition of your teeth becomes a low priority.

Later, when treatment is under way it is very upsetting to find that some of the troublesome side effects could have been avoided and that they remain a problem well after the fear and danger is over.

Extensive surgery and radiotherapy to head and neck trigger side effects such as a sore dry mouth and swollen, bleeding gums which can quickly lead to serious dental decay and all that goes with it. It is much better to be aware and try to avoid and manage these effects. Your dentist and hygienist should be part of a wider team to ease you through.

Of course every case is different and yours would be treated individually but in general, surgery and radiotherapy combined leads to a sore and dry mouth because of its effect on the salivary glands. Radiotherapy can damage teeth directly.

There is a strong temptation to drink sweet drinks and sugary soft foods while cleaning your mouth can be uncomfortable. Sugars in your mouth at this time can allow the bacteria to decay teeth very quickly, especially as the saliva is depleted and cannot wash over them as it normally would.

Your dentist and hygienist can help you with advice on special cleaning techniques and other aids such as artificial saliva and by careful monitoring help you to avoid problems and unnecessary discomfort.

A last word on teeth from Carol

THERE are dangers in a dry mouth because insufficent saliva can cause tooth decay and increase the risk of mouth infection.

You should try and sip sugar-free liquids frequently, avoiding caffeine and alcohol and chew sugarless gum or sugar-free boiled sweets.

I find Biotene Dry Mouth Care products help me, but you should ask your doctor's advice first. They produce an oral balance saliva replacement gel, a dry mouth care mouthwash, an advanced oral hygiene dry mouth toothpaste and an antibacterial dry mouth gum.

CHAPTER FIVE

Ann's Therapists

THE next chapter is devoted to consultants and practitioners who have supported me on my journey.

The articles on Reiki, Spiritual Healing, Hypnotherapy and Hypno Healing have been part of my life for many years. Christine Gould then introduced me more recently to Cymatherapy which I found very relaxing and interesting.

I have always believed in regular six monthly dental and dental hygiene visits, which are now even more important.

About six years ago I became aware of the importance of maintaining one's feet. And lastly there is Transference Healing which I find very uplifting spiritually, as well as helping me to stay positive when hiccups occur.

Dieticians are very important when it is an effort to think or do anything physically to help yourself regarding nutrition in the very early stages.

So, from head to toe, inside and out, I like to think that I am helping myself in the best way that I can. It helps me to throw myself into projects like this book and to thoroughly enjoy the experience.

For full details of where to find these consultants and practitioners, please refer to the Contacts & Referrals chapter at the back of the book.

Oral Health after Major Surgery

By Christine Duke, Dental Hygienist

THE period following major surgery in the mouth is very trying for the patient. Normally there is major discomfort and swelling after the procedure and one also has to cope with all the emotion generated by the seriousness of the disease. Good oral hygiene will speed healing and minimise complications.

Keeping your mouth clean after surgery is obviously very important but there are hurdles to overcome, the major one being apprehension about touching the site of the operation.

Immediately after surgery the best advice will be to use a chlorhexidine mouthwash such as Corsodyl. This may cause temporary staining of the teeth but the benefit far outweighs this disadvantage.

Once your surgeon has given assurance that there is good healing of the site then try to overcome any nervousness about touching this area. More harm will be done by leaving debris which can cause gum infection. It may feel more comfortable initially to use a cotton bud to gently clean the teeth but this does not have the same ability to remove debris so should be used for as short a time as possible, before using a small-headed soft brush.

The other main hurdle is loss of sensation which can be an on-going problem and is more difficult to deal with. Disclosing tablets may help to show where the plaque is and try to watch with a mirror where the toothbrush is going as it will be so hard to feel its position. Small circular movements at the gum line for several seconds on each tooth should remove all the debris. Whether you use a manual or an electric toothbrush will depend on personal preference. The importance of placing the bristles at the gum line is the same for all brushes. Bleeding from the gums may occur due to a build-up of plaque during the time that it has not been possible to clean thoroughly but this will gradually reduce as the plaque is more effectively removed.

There are other dental aids which may be useful such as a single tufted brush for reaching awkward areas and bottle brushes for cleaning between the teeth. Please visit your dentist as soon as you feel well enough and he or she can examine and advise on areas that need extra attention. And your hygienist will probably wish to see you more often during the year after surgery.

Christine works at the Amsel & Wilkins Dental Partnership, Banbury.

Podiatry

By Caroline L. Stead, BSc, DPodM, MChS
State Registered Chiropodist & Podiatrist

WHAT are podiatrists and what do they do? A podiatrist, or previous name chiropodist, has undertaken a three-year degree course in order to practise. The practitioner is then trained to diagnose and treat foot and related conditions concerning their client.

A podiatrist's scope of treatments

Podiatrists can treat foot conditions including straightforward callus and corn removal, verrucae treatments in all ages, flat feet in children and sports injuries in the adult. They can also help to maintain good foot health for the diabetic patient.

In today's society we have all become more health aware, in both treating ailments and in the prevention of health problems. And it is possible for a person with a foot ailment to self refer to a podiatrist without the involvement of the GP.

Advantages of podiatry treatment

A patient with a foot complaint may feel awkward and possibly embarrassed in seeing their GP. The podiatrist on consulting with the patient may be the first medical person to see the patient and therefore is able to help in diagnosing a possible underlying medical condition to their patient's foot problem. The podiatrist therefore is useful in a preventative healthcare role.

Once a foot complaint has been resolved clients often like to keep up with regular podiatry appointments and in many cases this has been found to be a satisfactory way of maintaining good foot health.

Caroline Stead consults in Podiatry and Chiropody at Northampton.

Transference Healing

Where does it all come from? Alexis Cartwright who lives in Sydney Australia has channelled the information and technology for Transference from the higher realms. Alexis is constantly anchoring and perfecting new aspects of this profound healing modality.

TRANSFERENCE is a seventh dimensional frequency healing and ascension process that delivers profound transformational results. It unites all new energy healing modalities within it and unites science with spirit.

It is suitable for all ages, conditions and illnesses and is remarkably effective and easily incorporated into your life. It works supportively alongside other traditional healing methods and receiving regular healings allows you to achieve and sustain a consistent level of health, wellness and spiritual growth through the Earth and human changes.

Human beings are not just physical in nature. We are complex multi-dimensional energetic beings, with a complex geometric, etheric blueprint underlying and sustaining us and regulating the automatic function of the body's self healing system.

Our etheric body, DNA, chemical and hormonal make up is quickly changing resulting in what we call Lightbody symptoms, such as: new illnesses, viruses, diseases, emotional and mental disorders, dissatisfaction, unexplained or increased severity of symptoms and in many cases ineffectiveness of traditional methods of treatment.

It works by using frequency and light to balance and repair the etheric fields that surround the body. The etheric fields hold the DNA patterns that directly influence all aspects of our being. Transference healing templates within us create a self-healing process that works on levels and planes. The procedures of Transference raise our frequency and bring about a cellular rejuvenation, which can have a deep healing effect. Transference uses colour, sound, planetary energies, sacred symbols, sacred geometry, templates, master rays, the elements, crystal frequencies, shamanic energies and crystal essences within its process.

What will you experience? You will find a Transference session to be extremely relaxing, heartfelt and a genuinely healing experience.

For more information please contact Sandy Genna Reygan on 01933 224733 email reygan11@onetel.net

Spiritual Healing

SPIRITUAL healing is an ancient therapy that has been practised throughout history. According to the Prince of Wales Foundation for Integrated Health, healing is one of the 16 most widely used therapies in all major civilisations and cultures.

Many people confuse Spiritual Healing and Spiritualism. They are not the same. Spiritual Healing is not connected to any specific religion and is compatible with all beliefs. The word 'spiritual' refers to the quality of spirituality implicit in the healing process.

Spirit is within us and animals too. It reflects our vitality and state of mental, emotional and physical well-being. When reference is made to someone or an animal being 'high spirited', this suggests they are in a state of high vitality whereas the opposite, 'low spirited', indicates lack of vitality.

The essence of spiritual healing is that practitioners tap into the divine or spiritual energy and act as a channel for the flow of healing energy to the recipient. The aim is to enhance energy thereby encouraging the body to self heal, utilising its own natural resources and become whole and well. Healing works on every aspect of the person to promote harmony of mind, body and spirit.

Practitioners channel energy through the hands from an external source to those who choose to receive spiritual healing. They either make direct contact with the person or place their hands close to, but not touching, the physical body. Energy may be channelled to a specific area or towards the whole body. It may be experienced in various ways such as heat, coolness, warmth, tingling, or a relaxed and comfortable feeling. Each person is unique and the sensations can vary for each treatment.

Healing is available under the auspices of the National Health Service in many hospitals, GP's surgeries and clinics. It is considered a safe and beneficial form of therapy irrespective of the medical diagnosis.

Spiritual Healing is completely natural and has no side effects. It may be given for any illness, psychological, emotional or physical condition and is regularly used alongside conventional medicine. As well as its value in relieving pain and restoring the body to its naturally balanced state, people have reported improved attitudes, clarity of thought and a better quality of daily life.

All healing is beneficial and usually a progressive process. Several treatments may be necessary before a change becomes obvious. Although many spontaneous recoveries are made, the benefits can sometimes be subtle and not in the way expected. Some may develop a different outlook on life regardless of their mental or physical condition and start to appreciate what they can do rather than what they can't. If someone is empowered to cope with their circumstances, their quality of life is enhanced.

Healing is helpful after major surgery, serious injury, trauma or the after effects of chemotherapy and radiotherapy. It also boosts the immune system, thus promoting feelings of improved well-being. When working with the terminally ill, healing helps induce a sense of peace to them and their loved ones.

Distant and absent healing is also very effective. Dedicated practitioners will regularly spend time channelling healing energy to those in need, regardless of whether the person is in the same room or miles away with similar positive responses.

After obtaining the permission of a vet, all these techniques can be applied to animals.

To find a qualified healer in your area contact: The National Federation of Spiritual Healers. Tel: (0845) 123 2777.

Cymatherapy

CYMATHERAPY is a combination of sound healing and magnetic therapy dedicated to restoring optimal good health and well-being. These combined cutting edge techniques are produced by the most advanced state-of-the-art healing technology. The Cyma 1000 acoustic instrument emits sounds programmed with biological messages, that the body assimilates to promote healing.

Throughout history the power of sound has been an integral part of ancient cultures through religion, magic or healing. It was fundamental to all primitive societies in a variety of ways such as chanting, drumming, toning, harmonic and choral singing, as lullabies, working songs, or to serenade a loved one.

In society today sound represents different things to each of us. It has been used to please and entertain, modify moods and control feelings, advance spiritual development and enhance awareness. For many people it is a natural accompaniment to daily life. There are many advantages when it is used with wisdom, knowledge and understanding. It can create a sense of balance and harmony, calm us, accelerate our energies or assist meditation.

Scientists recognise that the human body is a highly structured complex of rhythms and cyclic vibrations. When all aspects are collaboratively operating in harmony, including heartbeat, respiratory rhythms, blood pressure, pulse rate, hormonal levels, tissues and cells, then good health abounds. Similar to an orchestra, when all musicians play in harmony the result is pleasing. Conversely the effect of dissonant sounds is unfavourable to the ear.

During the past few years the power of sound, as a therapeutic modality, has increased especially in the field of medicine. Music therapy is regularly used to reduce stress, for pain management, in dentistry, delivery rooms and operating theatres, when dealing with the elderly and with those experiencing special needs and emotional issues. Ultrasound is another example. Healthcare practitioners regularly prescribe ultrasound to diagnose tumours, clean wounds, pulverise kidney stones and alleviate pain in sore muscles and backs.

All sounds have the ability to transmit energy through a process known as 'resonance'. Every part of the anatomy, the cells, organs and tissues have their own natural resonance or frequency. Each responds positively to sounds that vibrate in harmony with them. The opposite occurs when discordant sounds are perceived which can lead to harmful results.

Building on the science of Cymatics, 40 years of cutting edge research has culminated with technology taking energetic sound healing to a new level. Cymatics is the study of wave phenomena pioneered by the Swiss medical doctor and natural scientist, Hans Jenny. He spent 14 years conducting experiments of how sound manifests into form. The shapes and patterns that emerged using sand, powders, mercury, etc. from the effects of tones, music and vocal sound were filmed and recorded.

The implications of Dr. Jenny's work for healing and vibrational medicine were vast. If sounds could change substances what effect would they have on our cellular structure? This inspired others, including English osteopath

Peter Guy Manners, to explore how cells in an unhealthy body differ from the cells in a vibrant healthy one. It was from this research that Cymatherapy has evolved.

Cymatherapy delivers natural sound frequencies that restore unhealthy cells to their original healthy resonance. This vibrational technique aims to transform disturbed inner rhythms using sound pulsations transmitted by a hand held machine. It is placed over the area of the body to be treated and frequencies matching the cells in a healthy body are emitted.

The Cyma 1000 instrument offers a wide range of harmonious codes that produce precise combinations of frequencies and audible sound waves along with magnetic therapy, to synchronise the cells back to a natural healthy state of vibrational resonance.

The audible harmonious frequencies are combined with the Chinese Five-Element theory, the Meridian system, Chakras, energetic stem cells and hormones. Together they create an integrated mapping system of energetic healing for the sound pathways in the body.

This unique and revolutionary system works effectively on both animals and people and in America it is regularly used with horses and household pets.

Cymatherapy may be supportive in rebalancing the dissonant energies related to: addictions, anger, arthritis, irritable bowel syndrome, depression, digestive problems, dystonia, phobias, physical injuries, aches and pains and much more.

The Cymatherapy vibrational techniques have been reported to be effective for facial rejuvenation – non-surgical face-lifts. Many practitioners in America specialise in this procedure.

Case Studies

School Phobia:

Twelve-year-old Bobby had not attended school for four months despite intervention from the Educational Welfare Department and a supportive Mum who worked in the school system. Every morning Bobby complained of feeling sick, dizzy, with a headache and too ill to leave the house.

Medical examinations, scans, input from an Educational Psychologist and a worried mother saw no change in the situation. In desperation Mrs B took Bobby along for a consultation with Christine Gould.

Christine's background is in education working alongside youngsters exhibiting social, emotional and learning problems. Mrs B witnessed immediate changes in her son during and following the Cymatherapy. Upon leaving the clinic he was dancing along the street and returned to school the following morning and continues to attend everyday.

M.E.

Depleted of energy, depressed, and with nothing to look forward too, Ellie had virtually given up hope of ever feeling well. At the suggestion of her doctor she booked an appointment to see Christine Gould.

Having undertaken the suggested therapy to address psychological issues, Ellie was offered Cymatherapy for the physical symptoms. Initially the changes were subtle and after the fourth session Ellie felt that she had reclaimed her life. Full of enthusiasm and energy she is able to socialise and can make her own choices as to how she spends her days - very liberating.

Physical Injuries:

While decorating the outside of his house Peter, aged 47, fell off the ladder, hurt his right shoulder and was unable to lift his arm. After 15 minutes of Cymatherapy he was astonished to be free of pain with the use of his right arm restored.

At a recent health exhibition Malcolm was introduced to Cymatherapy. He is a keen cricketer in his mid 40s who has suffered with knee problems for many years. Intrigued by the Cyma 1000, he volunteered to be a subject for demonstration purposes. During the treatment Malcolm didn't perceive anything happening. Yet upon standing, he had complete ease and comfort in both knees.

For further information about Energetic Bioresonance Rebalancing and to locate a practitioner in your area consult: Christine Gould, Tel: (01604) 624515.

Hypnotherapy

By Christine Gould

HYPNOSIS has been practised for thousands of years and its therapeutic use dates back to primitive times. As long ago as 350BC Hippocrates, also known as 'the father of medicine,' acknowledged that the source of physical disease was linked to what went on in the mind. Plato stated that, "the cure of the part should not be attempted without the treatment of the whole and therefore, if the head and body are to be well, you must begin by curing the mind".

The general consensus of opinion is that hypnosis is an altered state of consciousness. It is a natural, safe and familiar process we all experience – often without even realising it. We go through hypnosis at least twice a day without being aware of it.

The word 'hypnosis' is derived from the Greek word 'hypnos', meaning 'sleep'. This implies that in hypnosis you are asleep when in actual fact you are not. As you enter hypnosis your state of consciousness changes to one of feeling relaxed, drowsy yet still awake, with enhanced awareness but still in control of your thoughts and actions. This altered state of consciousness is a natural phenomenon with no side effects.

We all spend time each day in hypnosis more often referred to as 'daydreaming'. Hypnosis is a state of altered consciousness not unconsciousness. It is when our thoughts drift from the present reality but operate on 'autopilot'. How many times have you travelled from one place to another and can't recall part of the journey? Or experienced time flying past while undertaking a routine activity like washing the dishes, knitting or ironing? We still remain alert, engaged, focussed and fully aware of what is going on and yet in an emergency can respond immediately and effectively.

A common myth about hypnosis is that it involves surrendering control, thus being made to do something against your will. However, the opposite is true. Hypnosis offers you the opportunity to tap into latent powers and exercise the ultimate in self-control.

Another myth worth dispelling is the depiction of hypnosis, often in movies and its association with pocket watches, trances and speaking in monotones. Contrary to this perception, in hypnosis you would never say or do anything against your personal beliefs or will.

Everyone who participates in a live entertainment show is a volunteer. They have willingly elected to co-operate with the stage hypnotist and have every intention of following their suggestions. Without exception all the volunteers are awake, aware of everything and in full control of their faculties. Should an emergency occur they would still be responsive, alert and most probably the first people to vacate the premises if necessary.

All hypnosis is self-hypnosis. For those who become conversant with techniques for self-hypnosis and take time to incorporate it into their daily lives the benefits are tremendous. By actively taking personal responsibility for your own well-being you can develop deep states of relaxation. In this way you can enhance personal awareness and accelerate your potential in all areas of life. It boosts vitality, promotes self-healing, focuses attention, expands awareness and harnesses inner resources. Like any skill, it requires practice and when you have mastered it you have a resource that is yours forever.

Hypnotherapy is one of the oldest and most respected medical practices known to humanity. It can be considered a type of preventative medicine, recognised for its value in the treatment of many conditions. With the recognition that the mind and body are closely related, the medical professions are increasingly recommending hypnotherapy and self-hypnosis to address a variety of behavioural, emotional and health problems.

This dynamic therapy empowers people to take responsibility for their own health and well-being by harnessing the power of their subconscious mind to resolve inner conflict and change existing or negative behaviour patterns.

An experienced hypnotherapist will skilfully guide the client into hypnosis enabling them access to their subconscious mind, which is the seat of all emotional and behavioural problems. Working co-operatively, changes can be made in accordance with the clients' desired outcomes. In effect, making the changes is similar to updating the programmes on a computer or reorganising your filing system.

Hypnotherapy is regularly used to manage acute and chronic pain, for burns, asthma, migraine, and with cancer patients to relieve the side effects of chemotherapy or radiotherapy. It can also help in the relief of many psychosomatic disorders as well as maximising potential in artistic, creative and sporting fields.

HypnoHealing is a specialised method that addresses health and physical problems. It works on the basis that the mind heals the body. Positive changes lead to positive outcomes and when the mind believes, the body responds accordingly. Only graduates of the world-renowned Atkinson-Ball College are trained in this technique.

Hypnotherapy is not just about problems. It is about achieving effortless change and getting in touch with why you are the way you are and becoming the person you really want to be – Your Ideal Self!

Answers to some frequently asked questions:

What is hypnosis?

A state of relaxation in which the client is very aware of what is going on and is in complete control at all times. While in hypnosis you would never say or do anything that you wouldn't normally do, whereas people who participate in live shows have volunteered to behave in an uninhibited manner.

Can anyone be hypnotised?

Yes, if they want to be.

Will I be asleep?

No. You will be aware of what is going on all the time and just feel relaxed.

Can I be forced to do anything against my will?

Emphatically - NO! The client is always in total control.

Are there any harmful side effects?

Definitely not because hypnosis is a natural phenomenon we all experience every day.

How does hypnotherapy differ from other therapies?

Many therapies are conducted on a conscious level whereas in hypnosis you bypass the conscious mind. This allows direct contact with your subconscious mind where existing or negative behaviour patterns can be changed and inner conflict resolved.

How many visits will I need?

Three to four sessions are generally sufficient and for more deep-rooted problems possibly five or six.

Christine Gould has been part of a multi-disciplinary team at the Pain Relief Clinic, Northampton General Hospital since 1992. Tel: (01604) 624515

Reiki

REIKI is the simplest way of harnessing the universal life force energy to stimulate the body's healing capacity. Whether you are fit and well, have a health issue or challenge in your life, Reiki provides a complete system of self-healing that you can readily implement in your daily life. After the training course, Reiki energy is instantly accessible forever. All you have to do is place one or both hands on yourself or others and the additional flow of energy is activated. Reiki is far more than a physical healing modality because it brings into balance all four aspects of self; mental, spiritual, emotional and physical.

Dr Mikao Usui rediscovered this ancient tradition of energy transmission through the hands over a century ago. He was a distinguished Japanese scholar of comparative religions on a quest to find out how the ancients healed. Eventually he accessed the formula from Sanskrit texts and following personal confirmation, named the system Reiki. It is compatible with all beliefs and has no religious connections.

Reiki is a Japanese word, pronounced 'ray-key', 'rei' means 'universal' and 'ki' 'life energy'. It is the vital life force, which permeates and nourishes all living forms – people, plants and animals.

Reiki energy accelerates the body's natural healing processes and is regularly used as a complement to traditional medicine and other therapies. With the right resources the body is capable of healing itself back to its original state thus restoring balance and harmony.

As the energy flows through you, the brain wave patterns change to the alpha state. This is the natural rhythm of the universe and similar to meditation thus slowing down the ageing process. It has also been scientifically demonstrated that the oxygen in the blood increases by up to 30 percent.

Many people report feeling a deep sense of relaxation, warmth, tingling or chill during a Reiki treatment whereas others experience subtle sensations or, maybe, nothing at all. The effects may be felt physically or they may bring about a change of attitude, inspirational thoughts, creative insights, or solutions to challenging situations.

Reiki amplifies the biological intelligence that promotes the body's resources to heal a cut finger, mend a broken bone, regulate bodily functions, or assist the lungs to breathe. It reduces stress and tension, relieves pain and discomfort, while inducing inner calm, relaxation and renewed enthusiasm for life.

It is a valuable first-aid tool, which can be used at any time whether at home, work, or leisure simply by engaging one or both hands upon yourself, or others. In an emergency there is evidence of rapid physical healing, manifested by burns that do not blister, pain relief, a reduction of swelling, the cessation of bleeding and bruises that tend to fade overnight. An additional bonus is the ability to maintain a sense of calm and emotional stability.

This effective, holistic hands-on-healing system is available to everyone. There are no pre-requisites or academic requirements needed to attend the basic course of Reiki training. The system is very straightforward and easy to learn. This is evident by the fact that children as young as seven years old can attend the class at the discretion of the teacher.

The Basic Reiki Level I, Training Course takes place from Friday evening to Sunday evening. During the three day seminar, you will receive four attunements, learn the 12 essential hand positions used in a Reiki treatment and be introduced to the metaphysical causation of illness and your circumstances. The body is a metaphor for your psyche and every condition and situation has a meaning. Powerful metaphysical insights are provided in accordance with the original teachings. By the end of the programme you will be equipped to use Reiki to help yourself, your friends, your family, pets and even plants!

The seminar also includes the history, philosophy and principles of Reiki leading to:

1. Improved Communication
2. Heightened Self-Awareness
3. Enhanced Relationships
4. Increased Self-Confidence
5. Personal Growth and Empowerment
6. Metaphysical Understanding
7. Stress Reduction
8. Certification
9. *Course Manual*
10. *Post Graduate Support*

In accordance with Dr Usui's teaching there are only two levels of Reiki. The basic training course Reiki Level I, requires making direct contact with your hands on yourself, others, animals or plants. At the optional Advanced Training Course, Reiki Level II, you learn how to project the energy over distance and absently using a proxy or by direct contact with increased potency of the energy. An additional bonus is that your telepathic gifts may flourish providing you with tools and techniques to develop your extra sensory perception.

Once you have undertaken training in this ancient hands-on-healing modality it is available to you for the rest of your life. You do not need any top ups or to make further financial investments. Regular classes and daily practice are unnecessary. Graduates of **Rei-ki Academy** have the privilege of being invited, at the discretion of the teacher, Christine Gould, to attend future seminars at no additional cost.

To learn more about the original Usui Shiki Ryoho tradition of Reiki in its purest form, contact Christine Gould at Rei-ki Academy. Tel. (01604) 624515.

CHAPTER SIX

Facing up to the world again

By Carol Dunstone

FEELING a little more confident after my Radiotherapy treatment, I decided to have some retail therapy with my sisters. We were celebrating my first shopping trip out into the big world and in spite of weight loss and hair thinning, I really felt the need to 'tart' myself up again – to make myself feel and look better.

We entered a large, well-known, department store and split up for about 20 minutes, heading in different directions. I made a beeline for the Cosmetics and Makeup counters. I still had the visible after effects of burning – black marks on my neck due to the radiation. And my speech was definitely not very articulate.

I couldn't pronounce 'g' or 'c' at all. Suddenly I felt very vulnerable without my two enthusiastic interpreters, Inga and Judy and I began to seize up.

I was on my own trying hard and I attempted to ask the assistant if I could look at the 'On Offer' display, set up at the back of the counter. She stared blankly at me, turned her back and proceeded to assist another customer.

I stood there in utter horror, in a sea of confusion. Something so simple had turned into a nightmare. Because of my strange inaudible speech noises and no doubt my rather swollen, black face, the woman probably thought I was drunk!

My confidence completely gone, I fled from the shop in tears.

It is so important for those who have had any facial surgery and scarring to be able to face the world again and for both men and women, there are many different ways, particularly with the aid of good cosmetics and expert advice.

Amway – helping people live better lives

By Sharon Harrison
External Affairs Manager, Amway UK.

A COLLEAGUE asked me to meet Carol and Ann and to hear about their aim of raising money for FACEFAX through publishing this book. Knowing that Amway UK has a budget for local community sponsorship, I wanted to see if we could help to support this venture.

When I met Carol and Ann I was struck by their zest, enthusiasm, and compassionate nature, despite everything they had been through. I was moved when Carol told me about her shopping trip to the beauty counter of a major department store and I could not imagine how she had felt about such a humiliating experience. The story may sound trivial to some but it must have been such a blow to the self-esteem of the glamorous lady who sat in front of me.

We discussed plans for the book, how it would help people who had been through the trauma of cancer and how they had both used their own experiences to describe the journey of recovery.

They told me that the great thing about the book was that it would enable people to feel better about themselves. Although Amway's major Corporate and Social Responsibility Programme in Europe is for UNICEF, United Nations Children's Fund, there remains room for us, like many other larger companies, to help the local community and to do it because it's the right thing to do. Amway's vision is 'helping people live better lives' and since the launch of our Global CSR project three years ago, we have raised $26million for children's charities.

As well as agreeing to fund the book's publication, we realised there was a synergy between Amway and the book. It includes contributions from therapists and other service providers outside the medical profession who could help people feel better and get easier access to services. In this way Amway, as a 'direct seller', fits in.

The beauty of buying Amway products is that they are sold to the consumer via direct selling. Instead of the customer going to a shop to buy their products, they can have an Amway representative call on them at a time that suits, order the products on their behalf and deliver them to the door. All our products have a 100 per cent satisfaction guarantee, so if you're not happy, you can have your money back! Our sales people are trained in the products and can discuss with you your needs, whether it's ladies' or men's skincare or food supplements to supplement your diet.

We have over 450 own brand products ranging from nutritional food supplements to home care cleaning products. What a lot of people don't know is that we manufacture all our own brands of personal care. Products such as hair care and body care ranges, skin care and colour cosmetics. They are all researched and developed at our own manufacturing plant together with nutritional food supplements for which the concentrates are grown on our own farms in California.

If you would like to browse the range of Amway products available, then click onto our website www.amway.co.uk If you'd like to be sent some product information or would like to be put in touch with an Amway representative in your area then you can contact Amway on 01908 629400 or email us at, infocenter-uk@amway.com

As a member of the UK's Direct Selling Association (DSA), we are proud to champion this industry which brings a personal level of service to shopping which, unfortunately these days is often missed when out in the high street. There are a whole host of direct sellers within the industry. They are all regulated by a strict Consumer Code of Practice offering higher levels of consumer protection to the shopper than those required by law and great products which can either be bought through a representative or direct from the web. You can access other direct sellers and their products via the DSA website: www.dsa.org.uk

Our small contribution of funding has made it possible for this book to be published. We are proud to have done so and hope that it raises awareness of the FACEFAX Association and its continual dedication to helping people to live full and rewarding lives.

CHAPTER SEVEN

Recipes for mouth cancer patients

*(Metric measures are rounded up
to match Imperial measures)*

Carol's tips

NUTRITION is the key to good health and vitality. To regain your full strength and optimum health, you need to eat well.

The best sources of protein are: MEAT, FISH, EGGS, CHEESE, MILK, YOGHURT and SOYA.

Bread, biscuits, rice, flour, cream, cereals, potato, nuts, chocolate, peas and lentils also contain some protein. Protein provides materials for tissue repair and growth.

The most concentrated sources of energy are fat, butter and oils. These can be used in cooking, on bread, vegetables, etc. Sugars, glucose, jam, honey and Lucozade are another valuable energy source.

An adequate intake of protein, calories and vitamin C is important. A high calorie intake is essential with a fluid diet to maintain body weight and provide energy for building new tissues.

Vitamin C is essential for healing and the health of skin and gums. Fluids rich in vitamin C are fresh, canned or frozen orange and grapefruit juice, Ribena and Rosehip Syrup. Take one glass of a vitamin C rich drink every day.

Vegetables should be part of a balanced diet. Supplementary drinks such as milk shakes, Build Up and Complan or Fortisips, which are drunk between meals, contribute substantial amounts of both protein and energy. These can also be used to replace meals when you have lost your appetite or are feeling unwell.

Try to have three good meals a day and at least one pint of milk each day. Cook food well and mash with fork or put in liquidizer with plenty of sauce or gravy to aid swallowing until chewing improves. Fluid feeds should be taken through a straw or sipped from a spoon or glass.

Take small frequent meals to ensure an adequate intake of calories and protein.

Some ideas:

- Liquidize or sieve soups – add milk or milk powder or double cream.
- Liquidize ordinary meals (meat, vegetables and potato) then mix with soup, gravy or milk until the required consistency has been obtained.
- Try baby foods.
- Oxo, Bovril and Marmite can be used as flavourings or mixed with boiled water as a drink.
- Use prepared sauce mixes and cook-in sauces.

- Milk puddings and custard may be managed if diluted with milk. They may be sweetened with glucose or sugar and fortified with milk powder, Complan, Build Up, evaporated milk or double cream to provide extra protein and calories

- Yoghurts, if necessary, can be thinned down with milk and taken as a drink, flavoured with pureed fruit or seedless jam. Ice cream and jelly are another alternative.

- In the early days of recovery, I found sauces invaluable and I still do. Soups are important and nutritious and organic soups are particularly good. Thin soups are perhaps easier when drunk from a mug. Pureed soups are excellent, especially if thick like a potage. It's often easier if soups have been liquidized as there is less chance of coughing and choking.

Try to use vegetables in season e.g. broccoli, tomatoes, spinach, garlic, sweet potatoes, potatoes, beans, peas, cauliflower, red peppers, aubergines, courgettes, carrots and greens, to name a but a few. They are good if steamed on top or baked in the oven. A sauce can be added to help swallowing. Eggs can be scrambled, poached or softly boiled and mashed up with a little butter, made into an omelette or eggy bread.

Recipe for eggy bread: Mix whole eggs and milk and season to taste. Whisk together with a fork. Dip slices of bread into mixture and coat. Fry both sides gently in olive oil or butter until golden brown.

Eating a variety of food remains important in order to provide a balanced diet.

Other tips and suggestions:
- Lentils and pulses can be added to dishes.
- Rice may be difficult for some.
- Mashed potato can be used as a carrier with other savoury foods. This has now become a major part of my staple diet.)
- Lots of sauces and gravies.
- Pineapple sucked in the mouth very gently helps to produce saliva and also fight off bad bacteria.
- Plenty of liquids like cold water and milk. I always carry a bottle of water with me, jokingly referred to as my *gin* bottle.
- Porridge or Ready Brek are excellent for breakfast.
- Mashed bananas.
- Stewed fruits, e.g. apples, pears, plums and gooseberry fool.
- Yoghurts and smoothies.

Ann's tips

HUNGER can be a challenge to overcome. Here are some suggestions to *fill the gap,* when allowed to eat and drink soft food.

- Porridge with active manuka honey has very good healing properties.
- Pureed dates.

- Pure chocolate melted in milk, any type of alternative milk or water.
- Pureed fruit with ice cream, yoghurt or sorbet.
- Various fruit jellies.
- Pureed carrot.
- Salmon mashed with a sauce.
- Minced chicken, turkey or lamb.
- Pilchards and sardines.
- Mashed potato, sweet potato and avocado.
- Add eggs to dishes for extra protein.

Juices

Contributed by Clare Castell

THE following six juices contain beta-carotene, vitamins C and E and Selenium, and can be drunk on a regular basis to provide all-round goodness – but don't forget to keep eating whole fruit and vegetables too. You can find high quantities of beta-carotene in whole oranges and vegetables, as well as dark green leafy vegetables.

Each recipe makes approximately one 8 fluid oz (230 ml) glass of juice. Adults can drink up to three glasses daily but do vary the juice combinations for maximum benefit. Drink diluted if you prefer. Juice each ingredient and then blend using a spoon.

1. 2 large carrots
    1 mango

2. 1 medium cantaloupe melon

3. 3 large carrots
   6 large spinach leaves

4. 1 nectarine
   1 peach

5. quarter sweet potato
   2 tomatoes
   2 large carrots

6. handful watercress
   2 large carrots
   quarter red bell pepper

Berry Booster

150 g (6 oz) raspberries
150 g (6 oz) blackberries
sparkling mineral water

Process all the fruit in the juicer. Add the mineral water to taste.

Surprise Juice

6 apricots
6 lychees
2 apples

Halve the apricots and remove stones. Peel the lychees and remove stones. Cut the apples into wedges. Process all the fruit in the juicer.

Wonder Juice

5 carrots
1 beetroot
4 watercress sprigs
1 clove garlic, peeled

Trim the carrots. Cut the beetroot into wedges. Process all the vegetables in the juicer.

Cabbage Juice

4 spinach leaves
4 carrots
7.5 cm (3 ins) wedge of green cabbage
quarter potato scrubbed

Form the spinach leaves into balls. Trim the carrots. Process all the vegetables in the juicer.

Pineapple Juice

2 pineapple rounds – 2.5 cm (1 in) thick
2 apples
1 mango

Remove the outer skin from the pineapple and cut the flesh into strips. Cut the apples into wedges. Peel the mango and remove the stone. Process all the fruit in the juicer.

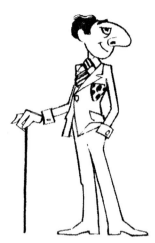

Elsa's Fruit Smoothie

Take a selection of fresh soft fruits such as mango, banana, peach or nectarine.

Liquidize with just enough fresh orange and apple juice to produce a thick puree.

Combine with a carton of Actimel, which sweetens and reduces acidity as well as making the drink easier to swallow.

Tip: If you can't be bothered to peel any fruit, just combine a commercial organic smoothie with Actimel for the same result.

Peggy's Soups

Avocado and Spinach Soup

2 avocado pears
half litre chicken stock
150 ml (quarter pint) cream or yoghurt
juice and rind of 1 lemon
300 g (12 oz) frozen or blanched spinach (well drained)
seasoning to taste

Scoop out avocado flesh.
Place in blender with rest of ingredients.

Blend until smooth.
Chill.

Tip: To keep colour of spinach, leave in fridge to last moment and serve in cold dishes.

Potage Bonne Femme

750 g (1.5 lbs) potatoes
3 large leeks, sliced
50 – 70 g (2 – 3 oz) butter
2 litres (3 pints) water or light chicken stock
Seasoning to taste

To garnish:
2 – 4 tbsp cream
parsley or chervil (chopped) and chives
Nut of butter

Melt butter in a large pan.
Add sliced leeks and cook gently until soft and shining.
Peel and dice potatoes.
Add to leeks and cook for 2 – 3 minutes.
Pour on stock, season, bring to boil and cook gently for 25 – 30 minutes.
Pass through coarse and then fine plate of vegetable mill. (DO NOT PUT IN LIQUIDIZER.)
Reheat, adjust seasoning and add butter, herbs and cream just before serving.

Potage Au Celeri

2 hearts of celery, washed and finely chopped
2 large potatoes, thinly sliced
75 g (3 oz) butter
2 pints vegetable or light chicken stock
150 ml (quarter pint) single cream

Cook celery gently in 50 g (2 oz) butter for 5 minutes.

Add the potatoes, stirring occasionally and cook for 5 minutes.

Add the stock, bring to the boil, season and simmer for 20 –30 minutes.

Pass mixture through a vegetable mill into a clean pan.

Reheat and adjust seasoning.

Just before serving add cream and whisk in 25g (1 oz) butter.

Creole Soup

1 large onion
25 g (1 oz) butter
1 small tin pimentos
2 tbsp plain flour
1 tin tomatoes
1 tsp tomato puree
paprika to taste
1.2 l (2 pints) chicken stock
1 dstsp horseradish sauce (optional)
1 tbsp cream

Chop onion finely and fry gently in butter until soft.

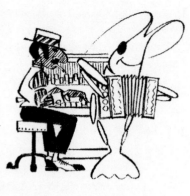

Add chopped peppers and cook 1 – 2 minutes.

Stir in flour and cook 1 – 2 minutes.

Add stock, tomatoes, tomato puree and seasoning.

Bring to boil and simmer 10 – 15 minutes.

Blend and then pass through a vegetable mill.

Adjust seasoning and add horseradish if desired.

Add a tablespoon of cream.

Tip: This is the last of Peggy's soups and might be a little too spicy for some people. It is also possible to use a liquidizer to blend the above ingredients.

Butternut Squash & Sweet Potato Soup

Contributed by Joy Ball. Serves 4

1 butternut squash, peeled, deseeded and diced

1 garlic clove, peeled and chopped

1 sweet potato, peeled and diced

4 tbsp chopped fresh parsley

2 carrots, trimmed, peeled and sliced

1 bunch radishes, trimmed and chopped (optional)

1 fennel bulb, trimmed and chopped

6 shallots, peeled and finely sliced

4-6 tbsp pumpkin seeds (optional)

1 wheat-free vegetable stock cube

Bring a large pan half-filled with water to the boil. Add the squash, sweet potato, carrots, fennel, shallots and stock cube.

Bring to the boil, then lower the heat and simmer for 10 to 12 minutes.

Remove from the heat and add garlic.

Allow to cool, and then strain the vegetables into a large bowl to keep the stock.

Add half the stock to the vegetables and blend in a food processor or with a hand-held blender to desired consistency.

Reheat the soup gently, adding more of the reserved stock if necessary.

Divide between warmed soup bowls and serve garnished with the parsley, radishes and pumpkin seeds.

Vegetable Soup

Contributed by Manjit Ohri

1 onion
vegetable oil for frying
1 carrot
1 potato
Small bundle broccoli
1 tsp mixed herbs
2 tbsp red lentils
1 vegetable stock cube
1.2 l (2 pints) boiling water
salt and pepper to taste

Chop and fry onion until brown.

Add mixed herbs, chopped vegetables and lentils.

Mix stock cube in boiling water and pour over the vegetables.

Cover and simmer until the vegetables are cooked.

Take off the heat and blend.

Season to taste.

Celery Soup

Contributed by Frankie Button

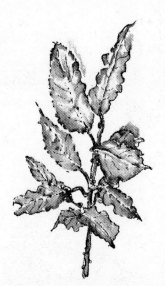

1 tbsp olive oil
1 onion finely chopped
Half a bay leaf
1 head of celery finely chopped
1 litre (1.5 pints) chicken or vegetable stock
pinch of mixed herbs
Seasoning

Heat the oil in a large saucepan, add the onions and soften without browning. Add celery, stock, bay leaf and seasoning. Cover and simmer for about 30 minutes or until vegetables are soft. This soup may be liquidized or not, as preferred.

Lentil Soup

Contributed by Frankie Button

1 tbsp sunflower oil
2 sticks celery chopped
3 carrots chopped
2 onions chopped
1 litre (1.5 pints) vegetable stock
1 tbsp tomato puree
225 grams (9 oz) red lentils
bouquet garni
3 rashers streaky bacon chopped (omit for vegetarians)

Heat the oil in saucepan and gently sauté the bacon, celery, carrots and onions for 4 to 5 minutes. Add other ingredients, bring to the boil and simmer gently for one hour or until lentils are soft. Puree or liquidize the soup and gently reheat.

Country Vegetable Soup

Contributed by Erika Takàcs. Serves 4

500 g (1 lb) carrots
500 g (1 lb) parsnips
500 g (1 lb) French beans
500 g (1 lb) small onions
500 g (1 lb) Kholrabi
1 clove garlic
500 g (1 lb) potatoes (optional)

Roux sauce:
2 to 3 tbsp oil
2 tbsp plain flour (or rice flour)
1 tsp red paprika

Cut all vegetables into little cubes.
Cook all ingredients in a stockpot until tender.
Season to taste and liquidize or leave chunky.
Heat oil in pan and fry flour until golden brown.
Take off the heat and add red paprika.
Mix roux well and add to soup.
Stir well and bring to boil, adding water according to thickness required.

May be served with shell pasta or croutons.

Chicken & Vegetable Soup

Contributed by Erika Takàcs

2 nice pieces of chicken breast
500 g (1 lb) carrots, sliced into round circles
250 g (half lb) parsnips, sliced into round circles
1 small onion (use whole)
3 bay leaves
1.8 litres (3 pints) water
a little milk
a good handful of fresh parsley
or 1 tbsp dry parsley
Vermicelli
Seasoning

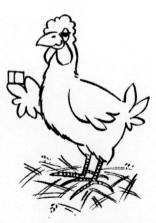

Cut chicken up into small strips, wash and cover with a little milk for about 15 mins. Wash off the milk.

Place all cleaned and chopped vegetables, bay leaves and chicken in a pot with 3 pints of water.

Cook slowly until everything is tender. You might have to top up the water.

Season to taste with salt and pepper. Remove onion and bay leaves.

The soup can be liquidized or left chunky.

In a separate pot boil 3 litres of water and when boiling drop in 3 rings of vermicelli pasta. When cooked, strain from water, rinse with cold water and serve with the soup.

Salads & Mousses

Snaffles Mousse

Contributed by Peggy Kimbell

250 g (10 oz) Philadelphia cream cheese
1 x 150 g (6 oz tin) Campbell's consommé – DO NOT CHILL
1 x 375 g (15 oz) tin Crosse and Blackwell consommé
garlic salt, pepper and curry paste.

Chill the Crosse and Blackwell consommé and the cheese.

DO NOT CHILL CAMPBELL'S CONSOMME.

Put the cheese, half of the Crosse and Blackwell consommé and all the Cambell's consommé in vegetable mill until smooth.

Add a quarter tsp of curry paste, garlic salt and pepper to taste.

Pour into ramekins and chill for 4 hours.

Decorate with remainder of chilled and chopped consommé or mock caviar or parsley.

Avocado Surprise

Contributed by Jane Garrard. Serves 4

2 avocados
juice of 1 lemon
125 g (5 oz) cream cheese
salt and ground pepper
50 g (2 oz) white Cheshire or white Stilton cheese, grated

Remove avocado flesh. Rub skins with lemon juice.

Mix avocado flesh with cream cheese and season to taste.

Place mixture back in skins and sprinkle with grated cheese.

Place under a medium to high grill and cook until cheese has melted.

Serve with walnut bread or rolls as a starter or main course.

Tip: Best with hard skins on Avocados.

Heulyn's Tabouleh Salad

Contributed by Heulyn Rayner

This salad should be made with cracked wheat (burghul), but cous-cous can be used instead. Tomatoes can be added. They make the salad a little mushier.

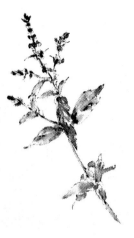

150 g (6 oz) couscous
1 medium sized onion finely chopped
3 tbsp parsley finely chopped
3 tbsp mint finely chopped
3 tbsp olive oil
Juice of 1 or more lemons, to taste
Salt and pepper

Empty the couscous onto a serving dish.

Cover with three quarters of a pint of boiling water into which you have mixed a tsp of salt.

After a few minutes, fluff up with a fork so that each grain is loose.

Mix with the remaining ingredients and allow to stand for an hour or two before serving.

Heulyn's Egg Mousse

Contributed by Heulyn Rayner

6 eggs
1 tbsp cream or crème fraiche

3-4 tbsp mayonnaise
1 small packet gelatine
2 small tins or 1 jar anchovies
1 tbsp chives
Half cucumber for garnish
seasoning to taste

Hard-boil the eggs, cool, peel and chop.

Mix together cream and mayonnaise.

Crush anchovies and chop chives, (reserving half of the chives for garnish).

Dissolve gelatine in a little hot water.

Stir all ingredients together and put in lightly oiled ring/mould. Refrigerate until set.

When turning out just before serving, decorate centre with diced cucumber and remaining chives.

Tip: The anchovies are quite salty so seasoning with salt is not recommended.

Judy's Broccoli & Apple Puree

*A wonderfully nutritious dish
contributed by Judy Shephard*

2 broccoli heads trimmed and cut into small florets
1 dessert apple quartered and cored
Half lemon
1 tbsp olive oil
2 shallots (or 1 onion) coarsely chopped
150 ml (quarter pint) apple juice
300 ml (half pint) chicken stock

1tbsp double cream
quarter tsp cinnamon
Salt and freshly ground pepper.

Steam the broccoli florets until very soft (about 15 minutes.) Set the broccoli aside.

Reserve 4 thin slices of apple from an apple quarter for garnish and squeeze lemon juice over them to prevent from discolouring.

Peel remaining apple pieces and cut into thin slices.

Put oil in a heavy frying pan over medium heat, add the shallots and cook until they start to look transparent, stir in peeled apple slices, apple juice, stock and bring the liquid to the boil.

Reduce heat and stir until apples are soft, stir in broccoli (reserving 2 florets for garnish) and heat through.

Put the broccoli/apple mixture into a food processor, add cream, cinnamon, salt and pepper, and puree until smooth.

Serve the puree immediately with the reserved broccoli florets and apple slices.

Sauces & Gravies

Creamy White Sauce

This recipe makes 300 ml (half pint)
and has a million uses in the kitchen.

50 g (2 oz) butter
salt and freshly ground pepper

1 skinned, finely chopped clove garlic
1 rounded tbsp flour
Freshly grated nutmeg
300 ml (half pint) milk
1 rounded tbsp finely chopped parsley (optional)

Melt the butter in a saucepan.
Add finely chopped garlic and flour.
Cook for 2 – 3 minutes, stirring continuously.
Gradually add the milk, beating it in as you go.
Let the sauce boil for a minute, still stirring.
Remove from heat.
Season to taste with salt, pepper, nutmeg and just before serving, stir in the finely chopped parsley.

Carol's comment: parsley is optional – omit it if it creates irritation at the back of the throat.

Onion Gravy

2 tbsp dripping or 3 tbsp sunflower oil (much nicer with dripping!)
3 onions – skinned and thinly sliced
1 rounded tbsp plain flour
600 ml (1 pint) chicken or vegetable stock
A few drops of gravy browning if liked

Melt the dripping and onions (if using oil, heat in saucepan before adding onions).
Sauté for 5 – 7 minutes until soft and transparent.

Stir in the flour and cook gently for about two more minutes.

Gradually add stock, stirring all the time until gravy boils.

Stir in gravy browning if you are using it.

Carol's comment: Delicious with toad-in-the-hole.

Savoury Lemon Sauce

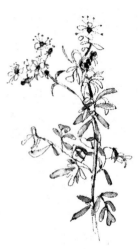

1 onion peeled and finely chopped
4 tbsp dry white wine
Juice of half lemon
1 tbsp finely chopped parsley
50 ml (2 fluid oz) chicken stock
50 g (2 oz) butter cut into pieces

Put the onion into a saucepan together with the wine and chicken stock.

Bring to a gentle simmering point and continue simmering in an uncovered saucepan until the liquid has reduced by half and the onion is soft.

Whisk in the butter a piece at a time and finally whisk in lemon juice.

Make sure that the liquid does not boil after the butter is added.

Just before serving, whisk in the chopped parsley.

Carol's comment: this sauce can be liquidized and is excellent with all grilled fish, meat and chicken and steamed vegetables.

Main Courses

Inga's Lemon Sole Florentine

Contributed by Inga Sutton

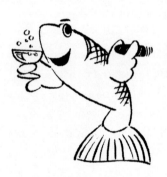

4 large lemon sole fillets
500 g (2.5 lb) spinach
Juice of half a lemon
25 g (1 oz) grated Parmesan cheese
35 g (1.5 oz) butter
35 g (1.5 oz) plain flour
450 ml (3 quarters pint) milk
salt and black pepper

Sprinkle the lemon sole with lemon juice, salt and pepper.

Fold the fillets in half crosswise and set aside.

Melt the butter in a saucepan; add the flour and cook, stirring for one minute.

Remove from heat and gradually blend in the milk, bring to the boil, stirring constantly until the sauce thickens.

Add seasoning to taste.

Wash the spinach, place in a saucepan with no added water (there is enough moisture on the leaves).

Cook for 2 minutes and drain well.

Stir half of the sauce mixture into the spinach and spoon into a shallow ovenproof dish.

Arrange the fillets on top and sprinkle with Parmesan.

Add the remainder of the sauce.

Bake in a preheated oven at 200c or 400f or gas 6 for 30 – 40 minutes.

Tip: Serve with freshly steamed vegetables and mashed potato.

Elsa's Loose Fish Pie

Contributed by Elsa Christie

2 pieces smoked haddock
1.5 litres (2 pints) milk
2 pieces cod
100 g (4 oz) butter
2 pieces fresh salmon
100 g (4 0z) plain flour
1 packet frozen prawns
half small packet frozen peas
1 kg (2.2 lbs) freshly boiled potatoes
100 g (4 oz) grated cheddar cheese
1 bay leaf
6 peppercorns

Poach fish for about five minutes in milk with bay leaf and peppercorns and leave it to cool in the milk.

Once cool, drain and reserve the milk for the sauce.

Flake the fish, taking care to remove all bones, peppercorns and bay leaf.

Place fish in shallow buttered oven proof dish.

Add peas and prawns, still frozen.

Melt the butter over a low heat and stir in flour until it thickens.

Gradually stir in the milk until the sauce thickens to a satisfactory consistency (you may have to add more milk if the sauce is too thick.)

Add grated cheese to sauce and stir until it melts.

Pour sauce over fish and peas and give it all a gentle stir.

Mash the potatoes with a little milk or cream and spread over the fish.

Dot with butter and place in fairly hot oven for about 20 minutes or until brown on top.

Tip: There is no need to add salt as the smoked fish and cheese are salty enough already. There should be enough sauce to keep the whole dish loose and moist. If it does not seem enough, make more before adding potatoes.

Carol's Creations

Lamb & Rosemary Stew

1.2 kg (3 lbs) lamb neck fillet (or stewing lamb) cut into 5 cm cubes

200 g (8 oz) new potatoes – halved (I sometimes add a sweet potato instead or as well)

300 ml (half pint) hot lamb or vegetable stock
2 tbsp olive oil
2 tbsp plain flour
4 tbsp freshly chopped rosemary
2 sliced red onions
1 small swede – chopped
1 small aubergine – chopped
1 tbsp tomato puree
large handful spinach (optional)

Heat the oil in a large pan over a medium heat.

Put the lamb in a bowl, add the flour and rosemary, season and toss to coat the meat.

Fry the lamb in batches for 5 minutes until browned all over.

Remove from the pan and set aside.

Add the onions, swede, aubergine and potatoes to the pan.

Fry for 10 minutes until golden brown.

Return the lamb to the pan with the tomato puree and stock.

Cover, bring to the boil and simmer for about 1 hour until the lamb is tender.

Remove lid and cook for a further 15 minutes to thicken the sauce.

Alternatively – put the lamb into a casserole dish and cover with foil.

Put into a pre-heated oven 150c and cook slowly for one and a half to two and a half hours.

Remove foil 15 minutes before end of cooking time.

Add Spinach and allow to wilt.

Tip: Serve with a dollop of natural yoghurt or cream or soured cream if desired. Freezes well.

Puddings

Frozen Pudding
Iced Orange And Apricot Mousse

for dinner/lunch party – serves 8

250 g (10 oz) apricots
juice of 2 oranges
Pared rind of 1 orange
3 eggs – separated
50 g (2 oz) sieved icing sugar
300 ml (half pint) double cream
3 – 4 tbsp orange liqueur

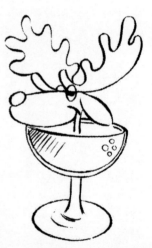

Put the apricots in a saucepan together with the orange juice and rind.

(Use potato peeler to pare the rind as thinly as possible).

Simmer gently until the apricots are soft. Rub apricots through a sieve to get a smooth puree. Leave to cool.

Whisk the egg yolks until stiff. Gradually whisk in sieved icing sugar – a spoonful at a time until you have a stiff meringue.

Whip the cream and orange liqueur together.

Fold the apricot puree into the whipped cream.

Fold the stiff egg yolk mixture into the apricot cream.

Using a metal spoon, fold the meringue mixture into the apricot mixture and place the whole thing in a large plastic container.

Seal and freeze.

Remove from freezer 20-25 minutes before serving and keep at room temperature.

Scoop out into a chilled bowl to serve.

Vanilla Custard

Makes 600 ml (1 pint)

600 ml (1 pint) milk
50 g (2 oz) caster sugar
4 large egg yolks
half tsp vanilla essence
1 tsp sieved corn flour

Put milk in a saucepan over a moderate heat.

Beat together the egg yolk, corn flour and caster sugar.

Beat a little of the hot milk into the yolk mixture and return to the milk in the saucepan.

Stir over a gently heat until the sauce coats the back of a wooden spoon sufficiently thickly for you to draw a line down the middle of the spoon with your finger.

Remove from heat and stir in vanilla essence.

Serve warm.

Carol's comments: this custard goes well with any steamed pudding and is the vital ingredient in any 'proper' trifle.

Jane's Apple Brulee

Contributed by Jane Kimbell

500 g (1 lb) cooking apples
50 g (2 oz) sugar
50 g (2 oz) brown sugar
large tub natural yoghurt or mixture of cream, yoghurt or crème fraiche

Peel apples and cook down to a pulp. Sweeten to taste and place in shallow dish.

Cover with yoghurt or cream mixture.

Sprinkle with brown sugar and leave in fridge overnight.

Pineapple Sorbet

1 average size pineapple
pared rind and juice of two lemons
1.5 pt / 1 litre water
2 egg whites
8 oz / 250g granulated sugar

Put the water, sugar and pared rind into a saucepan over a gentle heat until the sugar has dissolved completely.

Boil fast for five minutes.

Take the saucepan off the heat and stir in the lemon juice.

Leave to cool.

Cut the skin off the pineapple, put flesh into a liquidizer or food processor and blend to a smooth puree.

Strain the lemon syrup and stir into the pineapple puree.

Pour the mixture into a polythene container and put in the freezer for two – three hours.

Take container out of freezer and whisk pineapple mixture thoroughly.

Return to freezer for another two to three hours, bring out again and add the stiffly-beaten egg whites to the mixture and whisk thoroughly again.

Return mixture again to the fridge for one to three hours, then remove and beat and whisk for the final time.

Put sorbet mixture back in freezer until half an hour before serving (as you serve the main course). At the same time put the serving dish in the fridge so the sorbet remains firm when serving.

Serves 6 – 8.

Carol's tip: All the whisking and freezing really does make the sorbet light and gives it a good smooth texture.

Apricot Crumble

1 tin apricots in natural juice
75 g (3 oz) sugar – caster or granulated
200 g (8 oz) plain flour
100 g (4 oz) butter
Muesli (optional)

Put apricots in bottom of an ovenproof dish with some of the juice.

Make the crumble by mixing the flour and butter together in a bowl until you have a consistency resembling fine breadcrumbs.

Add sugar to the mixture as well as muesli if desired.

Pour the crumble mix over the apricots and place in a preheated oven 180c for about 45 minutes.

Tip: Delicious with custard and or ice cream.

Elsa's Slurpy Pudding

Sliced soft summer fruits (e.g. mango and oranges) or cold stewed fruit (e.g. rhubarb or apple)
Large carton of yoghurt or crème fraiche
Soft dark brown sugar

Place the fruit on a flattish dish or flan and cover it with the yoghurt or crème fraiche.

Sprinkle a generous amount of brown sugar over the top and set aside in the fridge, preferably overnight, to allow the sugar to sink down and flavour the whole dish.

Vanessa's Blueberry & Lavender Jelly

Contributed by Vanessa Kimbell

This delicious recipe has blueberries, which are full of antioxidants, and the cheese provides calcium, while the lavender lifts the spirits.

4/5 stems fresh lavender or 1 teaspoon of dried lavender
600 ml (1 pint) blueberry juice
mascarpone cheese
5 leaves of gelatine

Infuse the lavender and blueberry juice, warming gently – be careful not to boil.

Leave for between 30 minutes and 8 hours depending on how strong you like the lavender to be. Strain.

Warm the blueberry and lavender infusion and add gelatine, following manufacturer's instructions.

Pour into 4 pretty glasses and chill in fridge until set.

When set, put a large dollop of mascarpone cheese on top and decorate with fresh lavender.

Serve chilled.

David's Gingerbread Delight

Contributed by a FACEFAX member

Enough for one 900 g (2 lb) loaf

100 g (4 oz) soft light brown sugar
75 g (3oz) soft margarine
75 g (3 oz) golden syrup
75 g (3 oz) black treacle
105 ml (7 tbsp) semi-skimmed milk
1 beaten egg
150 g (6 oz) gluten free plain flour
50 g (2 oz) gram flour
Pinch of salt
10 ml (2 tsp) ground ginger

7.5 ml (1.5 tsp) gluten free baking powder
5 ml (1 tsp) ground cinnamon

Preheat the oven to 160c/325f/gas 3.

Lightly grease and line a 900 g (2 lb) loaf tin.

Place the sugar, margarine, syrup and treacle in a saucepan and heat gently until melted and blended, stirring occasionally.

Remove the pan from the heat, leave to cool slightly, and then mix in the milk and egg.

Mix the flours, salt, spices and baking powder in a large bowl.

Make a well in the centre, pour in the liquid mixture and beat well.

Pour the contents of the mixture into the prepared loaf tin and bake for one to one and a quarter hours until firm to the touch and lightly browned.

Allow to cool in the tin for a few minutes, then turn out onto a rack to cool completely.

Store in an airtight container.

CHAPTER EIGHT

Contacts & Referrals

THIS chapter lists the contact numbers, addresses and websites for therapists, medical specialists and products mentioned in this book, along with other useful numbers and websites connected with these particular areas.

Please note that clients are advised to seek medical attention before making an appointment to see a complementary or alternative therapist.

Allergies:

For information on the York Test for allergies contact www.yorktest.com

Arnica Gel:

For information on this massage gel, www.qvcuk.com The order line is 0800 504030.

Beauty & Nutritional Products:

Amway UK has numerous helpful products. Website: www.amway.co.uk. To receive product information or to contact a representative in your area, Tel. (01908) 629400 or email: infocenter-uk@amway.com

Coconut Oil:

Details of this nutritious oil at Coconut Connections, www.coconut-connections.com

Counselling Therapy:

Yvonne Miller, Dip Cou Studies, Dip NLP E.M.D.R. Therapy. Tel (07940) 544042.

Cymatherapy:

For further information about Energetic Bioresonance Rebalancing and to locate a practitioner in your area consult Christine Gould, Cymatherapy Representative in the United Kingdom.

Tel (01604) 624515 www.christinegould.com www.cymatherapy.com

Dentistry:

We can recommend
- Amsel & Wilkins Dental Partnership, 26 High Street, Banbury, Oxon, OX16 SEG, Tel: (01295) 253581.

- Waterhouse Dental Practice, 24 East Park Parade, Kettering Road, Northampton, NN1 4LB. Tel (01604) 638102

Diet:

World Cancer Research has a good deal of information on diet and health guidelines for Cancer Prevention: www.wcrf-uk.org

Dry Mouth care Products:

Biotène dry mouth care mouthwash.
Biotène oral balance saliva replacement gel.
Biotène oral dry mouth toothpaste.
Biotène anti-bacterial dry mouth gum.

Hairdressing:

We can recommend
- Sam Murphy, freelance hairdresser. Tel: 07866 375880.
- Windmills Ladies & Gents Hairdressing Salon, 53c Main, Road, Duston, Northampton, NN5 6JN. Tel. (01604) 757771.
- Lynda Evans, Tel. (01604) 760360.

Health & Beauty Therapy:

Michele's at Windmills Salon, Duston. Tels: 07939 580023 and (01604) 757771.

Hypnotherapy:

- Christine Gould is part of a multi-disciplinary team at the Pain Relief Clinic, Northampton General Hospital. Tel: (01604) 624515. www.christinegould.com
- Charles Callis is a consultant working from his own clinic at Wellingborough. Tel: (01933) 224454 www.hypno-corp.org www.abc-hypnptherapy.co.

Nails:

Michele Pennington, B10 Sculpture Gel Nail Studio at Windmills Salon, Duston. Tel. 0772 0715772 and (01604) 757771.

Nursing:

Macmillan Specialist Nurse Service. Contact Pauline Feast, ENT Outpatients Dept, Northampton General Hospital NHS Trust, Cliftonville, Northampton NN1 5BD.

www.aboutmyhealth.org-(link)
www.macmillancancersupport.uk
wwwcancerbackup.org.uk
www.cancerhelp.org.uk

Nutrition:

Kay Davies, Nutrition & Dietetics Dept, Billing House, Northampton General Hospital. Tel: (01604) 634700.

Oncology:

- Pauline Feast, Macmillan Nurse head and neck specialist, Head and Neck Unit, ENT Outpatient's Department, Cliftonville, Northampton, NN1 5BD. Direct line (01604) 523860. Email: paulinefeast@ngh.uk
- Macmillan Cancer Information & Support Centre, Northamptonshire Centre for Oncology, Northampton General Hospital, Cliftonville, Northampton, NN1 5BD. Tel. (01604) 544211.
- Oncology Hair Care Adviser: Tel. (01604) 544486.
- Macmillan Cancer Line: Freephone: 0808 808 2020. Email: cancerline@macmillan.org.uk. Website: www.macmillan.org.uk
- Cancer BACUP. For information, help and support about all aspects of cancer. Freephone: 0808 800 1234. www.cancerbacup.org.uk
- Rarer Cancers Forum. www.rarercancers.org.uk
- Look Good – Feel Better. Helping to improve the quality of life for women living with cancer.
  At Oxford. Maggie's Cancer Information, Churchill Hospital. Tel. (01865) 225690.
  At Cambridge, Addenbrookes Hospital. Tel. (01223) 216313.
- Changing Faces, London. The way you face disfigurement. Email: info@changingfaces.co.uk Website: www.changingfaces.co

Organic and other Health Foods:

Special dietary needs at Daily Bread Co-operative, The Old Laundry, Bedford Rd, Northampton NN4 7AD. Tel. (01604) 621531.

Physiotherapy:

The Physiotherapy Department, Northampton General Hospital. Tel. (01604) 545557.

Podiatry & Chiropody:

Caroline Stead, BSc, DPodM, MChS is a State registered Podiatrist and consults at 1 Boughton Green Road, Northampton. Tel: (01604) 791220.

Reflexology & Aromatherapy Massage:

Jo Wiles, Reflexologist AOR, Aromatherapist ITEC at Windmills Salon, Duston. Tels: (01604) 757771 and 07870 625017.

Reiki Healing:

To learn more, contact: Christine Gould at Rei-ki Academy, Tel (01604) 624515.   www.christinegould.com

Research:

World Cancer research Fund (WCRF UK), 19 Harley Street, London W1G 9QJ. Tel: 02073434205. Fax: 02073434201.

Speech & Language Therapy:

Contact Speech and Language Therapy Department, Northampton General Hospital. Tel: (01604) 545737. Leonie Bird and Elaine Coker.

Spiritual Healing:

The National Federation of Spiritual Healers, Old Manor Farm Studio, Church Street, Sunbury on Thames, Middlesex, TW16 6RG, Tel: (0845) 123 2777. Fax 01932779648. www.nfsh.org.uk

Swedish Body Massage:

Vicki Barber, I.I.H.H.T trained in Swedish Body Massage. Tel: (01604) 409013.

Therapeutic & Aromatherapy Massage and Reflexology:

Ilona Cydejko, MGCP, ITEC, MNSH. Tel: 01604) 402708.

Transference Healing:

Contact Sandy Genna Reygan, Tel: (01933) 224733, email reygan11@onetel.net

For in depth information, www.transferencehealing. com

CHAPTER NINE
The FACEFAX Association

THE FACEFAX Association aims to raise the profile of maxillofacial units and the treatment of face, head, and neck cancers by representing patients and treatment units everywhere. It is a central organising body that provides direction and acts as a central source for co-ordinating information and raising charitable funds.

It arranges the sharing of knowledge nationwide on head and neck surgery, in both the public and professional sectors. It makes maximum use of all forms of publicity including posters, direct mailing and the national media.

FACEFAX aims to promote the self-awareness and self-examination that leads to early diagnosis, referral and treatment. It will do this by networking information through local support groups attached to all NHS maxillofacial surgical units and any other NHS surgical units treating head and neck cancer.

The association supports patients by promoting their physical and mental health before surgery and during rehabilitation. This can be done through education, practical advice and, in specialised cases, financial assistance. Patients may be given further aid after maxillofacial surgery, chemotherapy or radiotherapy from facilities, support services and equipment not normally provided by the NHS.

Carers in the family are supported with advice and education on how to apply specialised care techniques. In exceptional circumstances, approved by the trustees, they will be offered limited financial aid when none is available from other sources.

To support these aims, FACEFAX produces leaflets and booklets for patients or their advisors to help those who have had maxillofacial surgery, particularly reconstructive surgery. This support is directly available to support groups nationwide, which will in turn, support the patients and carers in their local group.

Where necessary, FACEFAX will help provide domestic or personal equipment to aid the patient in eating or communicating and in their physical well-being. Such equipment may be designed and manufactured if suitable specialised equipment is not available from other sources.

The FACEFAX Association can provide specialist counselling, training and hands-on instruction for carers, supported with suitable documentation. And in extreme cases it can provide limited financial aid if specified by the trustees to help local support groups operate satisfactorily.

On the professional front, FACEFAX can enable staff at maxillofacial units to further their education and provide further research into treatment. It will aim to motivate and promote research into prevention, treatment and aftercare, together with the supply of specialised equipment.

This will be achieved by providing funds, when available, for educating and training medical or surgical personnel. This would be in specialised subjects or techniques that help maxillofacial patients and are not normally covered. And by funding selected research projects and the acquisition of specialised equipment.

For more information visit our website: www.facefax. org.uk

Notes

Notes

Notes

Notes

Printed in the United Kingdom
by Lightning Source UK Ltd.
114893UKS00001B/76-519